# Praise for *Oh Sis, You're Pregnant!*

"Finally! This gem of a book answers our questions about pregnancy and childbirth AND is culturally sensitive and socially aware. Everyone needs a 'Sis' like Shanicia Boswell. She is a fun, energetic, knowledgeable, and loving guide who takes the specific needs and concerns of Black parents seriously. I wish *Oh Sis, You're Pregnant!* was available during my pregnancies."

—Tatyana Ali, wife, mother, actress, singer, and filmmaker

"Black Pregnancy is a soul-filled journey to unveil some of creation's best work. This is a book that we all should have and a journey that birthed us all. I Love It."

—Anthony Hamilton, Grammy Award-winning singer, song writer, producer, actor, author, and father

"This book stands as the modern-day guide to birthing while Black. Women of color are in need of a book to help navigate the medical system as well as understanding how to take control of their pregnancy, overall health, and family's health. This book can be used as a nice compliment for any provider caring for birthing families of color."

—Angelina Ruffin-Alexander, certified nurse midwife and owner of Touch of Osun Midwifery Services

"Shanicia has written a book that focuses on what pregnancy is like for a Black woman. Pregnancy is more than what happens to our bodies during the nine months. Pregnancy is learning proper nutrition that benefits mom and baby. It's knowing healthy foods to eat while breastfeeding. Pregnancy for Black women is knowing what diseases we are more prone to develop based on the food we take into our bodies. This information will benefit mothers for generations to come."

—Chef Ahki Taylor, celebrity chef, wellness guru, and author

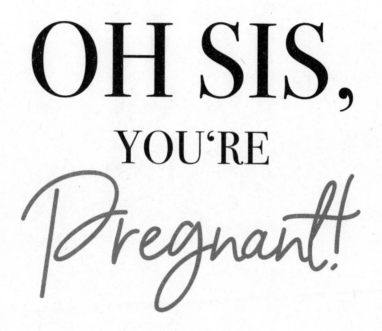

# OH SIS,
## YOU'RE
### Pregnant!

# OH SIS, YOU'RE

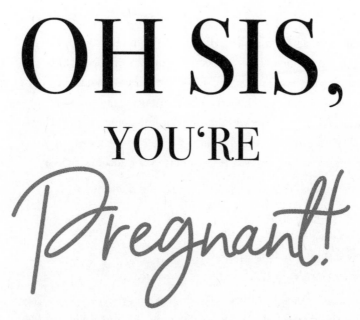

*Pregnant!*

## The Ultimate Guide to Black Pregnancy & Childbirth

### Shanicia Boswell

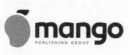
mango
PUBLISHING GROUP

CORAL GABLES

**The author is not a medical provider. Please discuss your birth options with your OB, midwife, or doula.**

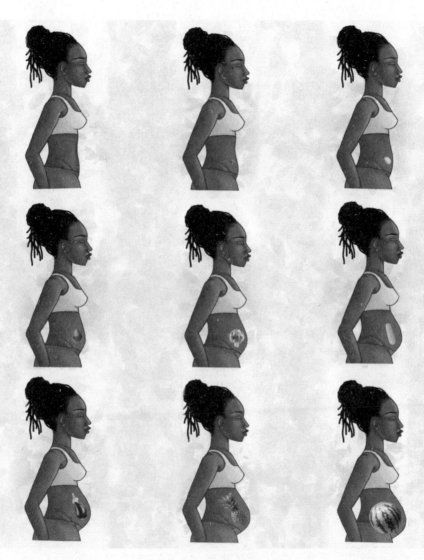

Artwork by Alexandre Keto

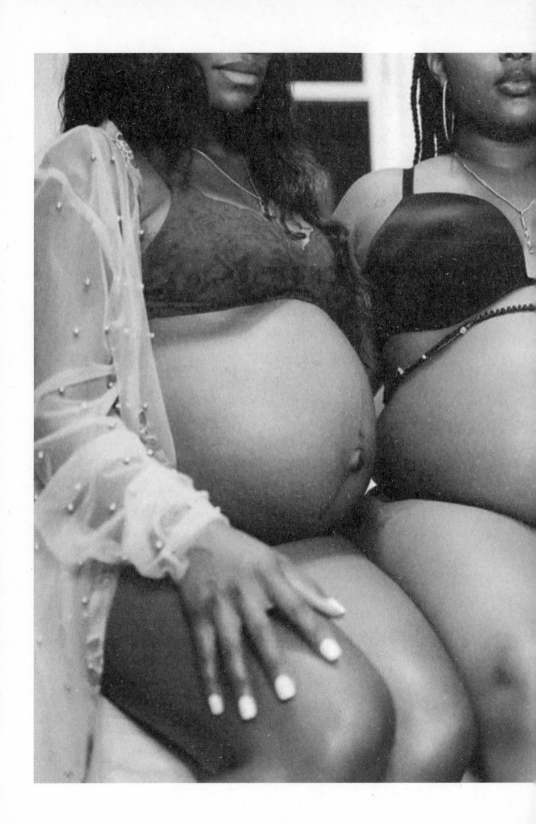

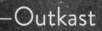

Yeah, this one right here goes out
To all the baby's mamas' mamas
Mamas, mamas, baby mamas' mamas
Yeah, go like this.

—Outkast

# Table of Contents

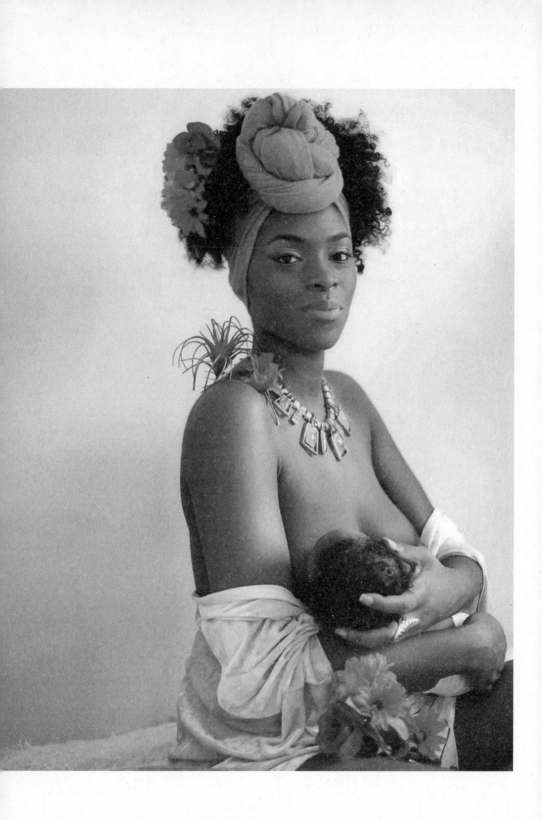

# Introduction

# Motherhood Is the New Wave

*We delight in the beauty of the butterfly, but rarely admit the changes it has gone through to achieve that beauty.*

—Maya Angelou

**Becoming pregnant at twenty-two years** old felt like accidently getting knocked up at sixteen in high school. Instead of walking the long hallways, bypassing judgmental eyes of my few hundred peers, I was trying to find creative ways to post on social media to hide my ever-growing baby bump. I was not ready to share with the world that I, someone that had not even fully broken down the doors of adulthood, was about to be somebody's mama. At twenty-two years old I had landed a successful job as the assistant to a person who was a lot more accomplished than me. At least I had my own office. I rented a hipster studio apartment in the middle of the city. Maybe because of my concern for the environment or because of the small paycheck that just barely allowed me to make student loan payment deadlines, I was economical and took the train instead of driving a car.

So, there I was, sitting on the toilet on Valentine's Day. It just so happened on the day of love that my breasts were unusually tender, and my period was not where it was supposed to be—in my underwear. As a responsible, sexually active woman, I always kept a few pregnancy tests under my bathroom sink. At this moment, I decided to take a test just to be sure. I did not think I was pregnant. I just needed the confirmation of that one little line to tell me to be patient and wait a few more days. Aunt Flo probably had plans of arriving unannounced in middle of the most painfully awkward situation. I peed confidently. I hummed a little tune as my fluids splashed onto the pregnancy test, and as I lifted that white stick from between my legs, I nearly rolled my eyes and yawned. Why did I waste a perfectly good pregnancy test to find out what I already knew?

There is this feeling you have when something catches you completely off guard, and you have no idea that there is even an inkling of a possibility that this could happen to you. You would think that I was the Virgin Mary sitting there taking a pregnancy test, and even she got pregnant. Those two faint blue lines popped up faster than I could blink. What happened to waiting two minutes? Those two minutes are extremely crucial: at least those discretionary minutes allow you the time to process this possibility of actually having a baby, since I clearly had not done this before. Regardless, there I was, sitting on the toilet naked, with a positive pregnancy test in my hand.

Shit.

And like any twenty-two-year-old, I called my best friend and screamed "*SHIT!*" so loud into the phone she probably still has nightmares about it. Lucky for me, my best friend lived only a few floors above in the same building. I put on my clothes, grabbed the pissy pregnancy test, and walked up to her apartment. Here is your first lesson: don't let anyone talk you into wrapping your pee-drenched pregnancy test in purple and pink tissue paper to hand to your boyfriend, who will probably freak out right along with you.

I will be honest; I was not too confident about what was ahead of me. Being a young Black millennial, I had not even accomplished my first goal of finishing college. I was currently on a sabbatical to figure out life. This was one of things I realized early on in my twenties—I had a certain privilege. Even as a Black woman, I had privilege. I had the privilege to take time off from college to "*find myself.*" And I had been working on it. I took a two-week trip to Egypt to connect with my ancestors. I got rid of my phone for three months, dyed my afro a weird combination of purple, orange, and red, and even converted to a religion. I had become the poster child for Black, privileged youth, squandering opportunities that my elders had fought so hard for me to have. Even I knew I had maybe gone too far left and had started to reel it back in. I dyed my hair back black, made the decision to loc it up, and landed a job in corporate America. I was looking for the American Dream before even realizing what my own dream was. I was trying to be my ancestor's wildest dreams without proper context. Did my ancestors really want me filing papers for eight hours a day? Probably not. They also did not want me pregnant at twenty-two either but here we were.

. . .

That was nearly a decade ago, and in these last few years so much has changed—most importantly, my mindset and outlook on life. Since that life-changing discovery of pregnancy, I have successfully mommed the hell out of my twenties and become an inspirational writer and entrepreneur who has dedicated her livelihood to uplifting and encouraging other Black mamas, as well as an advocate for self-care. I have also tanked a business, called off an engagement, hit rock bottom, and built myself back up. I did all of this with my child in tow.

What is my goal in writing this guidebook? My goal is to let other mothers know that you, yes you reading this book, YOU are perfectly imperfect. I want to cure you from the mom guilt you may be holding on to because your pregnancy did not happen the way you wanted it to. I want to make you laugh, maybe cry a little as you look toward your own experience and invoke a spiritual

"*Yasssssss sissss*" through the pages of this book. While there are similarities for many who are becoming mothers, regardless of race, color, religion, or culture, our experiences specifically as Black mamas are unique. I wear that knowledge as a proud badge of honor.

As the creator of *Black Moms Blog*, I am asked a lot: Why create a platform for only Black mothers and not all mothers? My answer is simple: *Black Moms Blog* is not just an online space for Black mothers. We have mothers of all races, women without children, grandmothers, fathers, and grandfathers who are members of our community. *Black Moms Blog* is a space within the already marginalized space of motherhood to positively reflect Black parenthood. We uplift Black mothers. We share our experiences through our eyes. We tell stories of our grandmother's advice and wisdom, lessons on hair care and how to deal with our children being the only Black faces in the room. This book is an extension of that narrative. It expresses the collective thoughts and practical experiences I have found to be helpful as a Black mother: dating, traveling, and living my best life while tackling the ebbs and flows of motherhood.

My overall mission here is to let you know that life does not have to stop because you chose to give birth. In fact, it is just beginning. There is something powerful in living life and knowing that your strength, not only as a Black woman but as a Black mother, is being seen by your daughters and your sons. We are rewriting the stories, changing the statistics, and creating a generation of children ahead of us that will know that because we did it, they can do it better. This is *The Ultimate Guide to Black Pregnancy and Motherhood*.

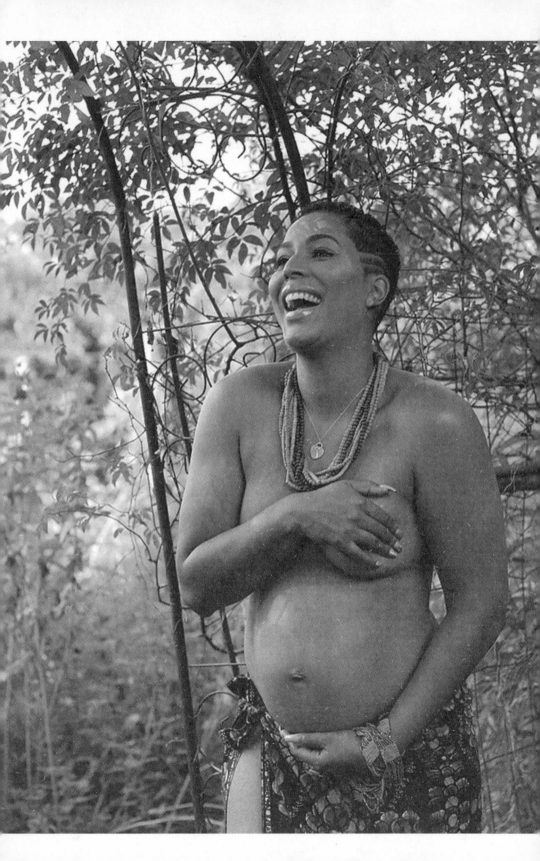

# Chapter One

# My Growing Belly Bump

*Becoming a mother
forced me to
have hope.*

—Nefertiti Austin

**Here is something you have** probably already discovered while pregnant: there are a ton of educational guides out there that will tell you when your baby grows from the size of a grape, to the size of an avocado, to the size of a watermelon. These guides probably come with adorable photos and let you know that your feet may bulge, your rings will no longer fit your fingers, and, lucky for us, our noses will change too. Oh yes, our noses will widen. You will learn about what is happening with your body, why your nipples darken, and about that strange line going down your belly. These books will spend chapters explaining all this to you. While this falls under the category of necessary information, I believe there is a wealth of more important knowledge you need to know about to actually prepare for the impending birth.

In the chapters that fill this book, I want to concentrate on topics that really will affect your life, Sis. I want to talk to you about why using your voice is important and how it relates to Black maternal health. I want to chat with you about the real, grown conversation you will have with your own mother about what is allowed and not allowed when you are giving birth. I want to walk you through getting your finances in order. Are you prepared for this? I especially want to chat to you about the changes that you will go through emotionally, how your friendship circles may evolve, and how to cope if you find yourself in the position of being a single mama. Throughout this book, I want to reach out and hold your hand. I believe that these topics are much more important. As a Black mother, I want to share my own experience to help prepare you for your birth.

Even still, I know how reassuring it is for you to know the size of your baby at four months versus six months and whether or not you should be excited that your breasts have magically gone up two cup sizes, so we will discuss some of that now too. All in one chapter. Then we can move on to some of the other topics that will help prepare your mind for motherhood. Bookmark this page and refer back to it throughout your pregnancy.

# The Science of Getting Pregnant

I want to let you in on a little-known fact—there are a lot of occurrences that have to take place in order for you to become pregnant. We seem to mystify pregnancy, but it is so necessary to understand exactly how pregnancy happens and how many important steps have to align in order for a woman to have a child. Pregnancy is no "accident." Your body and your partner's or donor's sperm have to come together at the perfect time to create a baby. Let's break down what happens leading up to the moments that your baby is formed.

Pregnancy can occur in many different ways. There is the traditional way, meaning a man and woman have sexual intercourse and he releases sperm into her vaginal canal resulting in pregnancy. In vitro fertilization (IVF) has become increasingly popular over the years. IVF is a method normally used by couples who are facing difficulties with conceiving. A woman takes medication, usually injected in shots over a period of time, which help stimulate the production of her eggs. The eggs are then removed by a needle inserted into the pelvic cavity and the eggs and sperm are joined in a laboratory. Once an embryo, or a multicellular organism, is formed, then the embryo is placed back into the woman's uterus where the pregnancy can continue. Intrauterine insemination, or IUI, is when a medical provider uses a catheter to insert sperm into a woman's vaginal canal, through the cervix, directly to the egg inside of the uterus. Lastly, there is the bootleg version of IUI otherwise known as "turkey basting." This is not recommended by doctors, but it is a method that is practiced, particularly by same-sex couples. Sperm, either from a donor or a sperm bank, or sometimes acquired by other methods, is collected in a cup then syringed into the turkey baster. The baster is inserted with a sperm-friendly lubricant and the sperm is injected into the vaginal canal. The woman lies flat with her legs in the air for ten minutes, so the sperm doesn't leak from the vagina. This is best done during ovulation and after orgasm so that the sperm has a better chance of entering the cervix to reach the egg in the uterus. A gentle reminder: if this method of achieving pregnancy is used, you can run the risk of infection or contracting an STI if the sperm is not properly tested.

# A Very Real Conversation on the Birds and the Bees

Do you remember your first "birds and the bees" conversation with your parents? It went something like this: The bees pollinate the flower. The birds hatch the egg. As an adult, I look at this wildly far-fetched account and am lost in the exact correlation of the bird and the bee. I understand that the bee pollinating the flower represents a man's sperm fertilizing a woman's egg and that the bird hatching the egg represents the woman giving birth, but who decided to join these two unrelated creatures in a sexual act? We are adults now. Let us put the hypotheticals to rest and have a very real conversation.

The first step of pregnancy is called fertilization. This is when a woman's egg and a man's sperm join together, usually in the woman's fallopian tube. Fun fact: the sperm carries half the genetic information for your baby. This includes, but isn't limited to, genes relating to hereditary diseases, stress, and even metabolism. If your kid ends up with a strange diet, you can blame their father!

When a man ejaculates inside of a woman, he releases roughly 300 million sperm inside of her vaginal canal. Immediately, this number of sperm is greatly reduced when millions of sperm flow out of the vagina or are killed by acidic pH levels in the vagina. During the few days that a woman is ovulating, her cervix is open, and the surviving sperm can enter and swim through thin and slippery cervical mucus. Consider this your body's way of encouraging pregnancy. The cervical mucus becomes watery during ovulation for this very reason—to help move the sperm along to the uterus along with muscle contractions that speed up the sperm's journey. Millions more sperm die by becoming stuck in the cervical folds or are killed by the woman's immune system, once again reducing the number of sperm that will possibly reach the egg. While looking for the uterus, the remaining few thousand sperm find themselves at a crossroads, with half choosing the wrong direction and heading toward the empty fallopian tube and the other half heading in the right direction, toward an egg to possibly fertilize. Inside of the fallopian tubes are tiny hair like fibers called cilia that push the egg through the tube. The sperm have to swim against this motion, and more sperm are lost by becoming trapped in the cilia. During this time, the sperm undergo a transformation due to the chemicals in the reproductive tract. This causes a surge of hyperactivity and the sperm swim faster toward the egg.

Of the original 300 million sperm, only a few dozen remain once the sperm reaches the egg. Our eggs are protected by a layer of cells called the corona radiata which the sperm has to push through only to reach another layer of protective cells called the zona pellucida. Once these protective cell layers are bypassed, the sperm attaches itself to specialized sperm receptors on the surface of the egg, causing digestive enzymes to be released from the sperm. This allows the sperm to burrow into the layer of the zona pellucida. The first sperm that makes it through fertilizes the egg. Usually only one sperm out of 300 million attaches to the egg cell membrane, and then the membrane hardens to keep out all other sperm that may be trying to attach to fertilize the egg. One sperm out of 300 million. Your pregnancy has a purpose, Sis. Don't ever forget that.

# What about Moms of Multiples?

If you are currently pregnant with twins or multiples, consider yourself a part of the special group of only 4 percent of births worldwide. The number of fraternal twins and multiples have actually increased due to more women seeking out fertility treatments to become pregnant. Other factors such as genetics, age, and location also affect the rate at which mothers birth multiples. Women from Africa, as well as older mothers, are more likely to birth fraternal twins. A mom of multiples is considered to be a hyper-ovulating woman, which is hereditary through the maternal line.

Keeping things simple, let's focus on the most common two types of multiples—identical and fraternal. Identical twins are called monozygotic, and fraternal twins are referred to as dizygotic. Mono, or one, means that only one zygote is formed, and di, or two, means two zygotes are formed. When the sperm implants the egg in a monozygotic pregnancy, the one zygote splits into two separate zygotes, basically creating a carbon copy of the first zygote. These two zygotes are either boy-boy or girl-girl. Monozygotic multiples have the exact same genes, all the way down to their biological gender. In a dizygotic pregnancy, two eggs are ovulated from the mother at the same time and fertilized by two different sperms from the father. These zygotes are completely different but just happen to be born at the same time. Their genes are not clones, so they have no closer relation than two siblings born five, ten, or even twenty years apart. These zygotes can be boy-boy, girl-girl, or boy-girl.

Understanding the scientific process of pregnancy is very important not only for your own benefit but so you have the information to pass on to your children as they become older. We also have to make pregnancy knowledge humanistic, relate it back to us as Black women, and take it out of its proverbial box. The science of pregnancy must be understood, and the visuals around childbirth and your growing baby bump are just as important. Think about it: how many times have you googled images of a growing belly bump and seen yourself? In this book, I want you to see yourself in every aspect, from the visuals to the education; everything you read here is intended to represent you. Let's explore what happens week by week during our pregnancy.

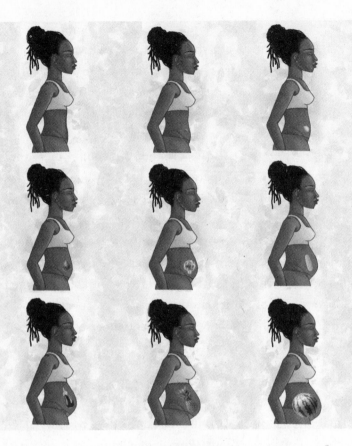

My Growing Belly Bump
Artwork by Alexandre Keto

**Week 4**: Your baby is the size of a poppy seed. You probably just found out that you are pregnant and are not experiencing intense pregnancy symptoms just yet. During this time, you may notice slight tenderness in your breasts, light cramping, and mood swings which could all be disguised as early signs of your menstrual cycle. Your little one is forming its amniotic sac, or bag of fluids, which will be the cozy home for your embryo for the next eight months. If you have not done so yet, pick up your prenatal vitamins!

Prenatal vitamins, or supplements, contain the right amount of nutrients and minerals needed for you and your baby. You can check with your medical provider about which vitamins are the best for you.

**Week 8**: Your baby is the size of a strawberry. By this point, mama, you may have better insight into your body's changes during pregnancy. You may be experiencing morning sickness and food aversions. While you are going through some major changes, so is your baby! Your tiny human is forming its eyes, nose, and lips, plus it has a heartbeat that is drumming away at around 150 to 170 times per minute—nearly twice as fast as your own. In the next two weeks, your doctor will perform genetic testing to make sure your baby is healthy. Your doctor may do an ultrasound to check you for placenta previa, which is when the placenta rests low and covers all or part of the cervix. This can cause vaginal bleeding and may result in a C-section birth.

**Week 12**: Your baby is the size of a lemon. Speaking of lemons, how are your pregnancy symptoms? You are nearing the end of your first trimester and some of your pregnancy symptoms should be starting to ease up a bit. You no longer look bloated and are beginning to look like the pregnant woman that you are. Wear it proudly! You and your babe still have six months to go. It is better to get used to the bump now rather than later. You may notice your nipples are starting to get larger and darker during week twelve. Your body is prepping early for breastfeeding. Don't be alarmed. Your little one is growing its white blood cells which will help fight off infections in the future, and at your next doctor's visit you should be able to hear your baby's heartbeat for the first time!

**Week 16**: Your baby is the size of an avocado. Have you felt your first kick yet? It is coming. Your baby has been working out! Your tiny avocado now weighs around four ounces and may need some sunglasses because his or her little eyes are in action and can experience sensitivity to light. The best part? Facial muscles are developing so your baby can squint, frown, and smile. Here's a tip: now is the time to start singing and talking to your little one. They can hear your voice! Mama, you may notice the horizontal line that has been forming on your belly start to darken. This is called the *linea nigra*, or "black line" in Latin. The *linea nigra* becomes hyperpigmented due to pregnancy hormones.

**Week 20**: Your baby is the size of an artichoke. You just hit your halfway mark, Mama! Those fluttery feelings in your belly may be gas...or it may be your little one doing somersaults. If you have not felt baby kicks yet, you are very close. You are also at the pregnancy stage where your baby's gender can be revealed if you choose the traditional ultrasound route. Your doc can also reveal your babe's gender earlier in pregnancy, around 12 weeks, if you choose to have a blood test done. Go ahead and prepare for your big gender reveal. As for you, Mama, you may notice an increase in your appetite. This is where that whole "eating for two" saying comes into play. Just remember, eating for two doesn't mean giving in *to all* of your cravings. Try to maintain a healthy diet, full of fruits and veggies for your growing baby and yourself.

**Week 24**: Your baby is the size of an ear of corn. Here is something you may find funny—your babe is still waiting to obtain their full melanated complexion. Right now, your babe has eyelashes, eyebrows, and hair, but is still lacking pigment, so their skin is transparent. Those juicy cheeks that you plan to kiss all day long also haven't formed yet, so sit tight. Your little fighter is weighing about one pound, and if you have been singing or talking to your belly on a regular basis, your babe can recognize their favorite songs. Mama, your belly button has probably popped, and you are sporting a cute outie right now. You may also notice some swelling in your fingers, knees, and ankles, so take it easy.

**Week 28**: Your baby is the size of an eggplant. You are now seven months pregnant and your baby is officially starting to get in a comfortable position for their grand entrance. For most moms, this means the baby is facing head down unless your little one is intending to come out breech, which means feet first. Don't worry, only 3 to 5 percent of babies born to term are breech births. Your baby is also dreaming about his or her life earthside too. During this stage of pregnancy, your little tike is experiencing different phases in the sleep cycle including REM (rapid eye movement) sleep, which induces dreams. If you see an ultrasound of your babe sticking their tongue out at you, it is okay to laugh! They may just be tasting amniotic fluid. Mama, your belly is growing more and more. This is the time to keep your hands off. No scratching! Massage shea and cocoa butters into the skin to keep your stretching skin from itching.

**Week 32**: Your baby is the size of a pineapple. At eight months pregnant, Mama, you only have one more month left to go! You may be experiencing Braxton Hicks contractions. Think of these as your body's unfriendly way of sending you irregular practice contractions to prepare you for your actual labor. If you haven't signed up for maternity photos, now may be the time to do it. Your belly should be full and sitting high, still perfect for capturing the moment in time of your pregnancy. Your little one is now about four pounds and sixteen inches long on average. He or she is moving a lot more frequently and practicing for their sleep cycle once they are born. Many mothers note that their little ones sleep on the same schedule in the first few weeks after birth as they did during those last weeks of pregnancy!

**Week 36**: Your baby is the size of a watermelon. You have officially made it to the ninth month of your pregnancy, and just like you, your baby is winding down and preparing for his or her birth. At this point, your little one is measuring around six pounds and eighteen inches. Your baby's skull bones are still soft so that it can fit through the birth canal, but its immune system and blood circulation system are fully formed and ready for the outside world. You may notice your belly drop during your last month of pregnancy due to your little one getting comfortable in your pelvic cavity to prepare for birth. You have nearly hit the finish line.

# A Quick Detour into Understanding Prenatal Vitamins

Prenatal vitamins are very important for women to take starting in their first trimester. For my mamas that are planning to become pregnant, you can start your prenatal vitamins a few months prior to pregnancy to make sure your body is in an optimal position to conceive. Prenatal vitamins help increase your iron and any nutrients you may be missing for a healthy pregnancy. They also increase your production of folic acid, which helps to prevent neural tube defects in your growing baby. To my fully healthy and nutritious mamas, I know that you may be inclined to skip out on the prenatals, but I encourage you to find ones that fit your lifestyle. It is true that nutritious foods and a healthy diet are the best way to supply your body with what it needs to support an ideal pregnancy, but because you need additional nutrients, you may be missing out on key supplements that prenatal vitamins supply. Key factors you want to check for when choosing a great prenatal vitamin are:

- Folic acid
- Iron
- Calcium
- Vitamin D
- Vitamin C
- Vitamin A
- Vitamin E
- B vitamins
- Zinc
- Iodine

Speak with your medical provider to find out which of these nutrients you may be deficient in, as this may result in the need for a prenatal vitamin that supplies more of one nutrient over another. The most common side effect of prenatal vitamins is constipation so make sure you are drinking lots of water throughout your day and eating more fiber. Check in with your doc to see if it's okay to also incorporate a stool softener if necessary.

This chapter is extremely important as you navigate through your pregnancy. I would also suggest taking monthly photos to track your growing baby bump. As your pregnancy continues, the initial changes in your body may not be that noticeable, but with photos you will be able to compare your changing pregnancy size visually. The average woman gains around twenty-five to thirty-five pounds during pregnancy. When talking about weight gain, it is extremely critical to discuss the factors in our community that can have a greater effect on our pregnancy health. Let's have a chat with a board-certified OB/GYN to learn about our risks and how diet and exercise can play a role in a healthier pregnancy.

# Chapter Two

# A Conversation with Dr. Heather Irobunda, MD, on Gestational Diabetes

*We need to do a better job of putting ourselves higher on our own "to do" list.*

—Our Forever First Lady,
Michelle Obama

**In the next few chapters,** we will discuss how your health as a pregnant Black woman can be compromised by the medical care provided to you during this delicate time. Even bigger though are the risks that can accompany you solely based on your genetics and demographic. Depending on pre-existing health conditions, age, lifestyle, and if you have had previous pregnancies, your pregnancy may be categorized as low risk or high risk. A low-risk pregnancy is defined as one that will need no medical intervention. Upwards of 92 percent of all pregnancies are considered low risk. A high-risk pregnancy, which occurs for 6 to 8 percent of all pregnant women, means that there is a greater risk to mother and baby during pregnancy and delivery, and that there is a strong possibility of the need for medical intervention.

For this particular conversation, I wanted to open up a dialogue with a seasoned medical provider who could offer her professional opinion on how certain conditions can have an effect on Black women during pregnancy. Dr. Heather Irobunda offers over eight years of experience in the medical field. She received her Bachelor of Arts from the University of Pennsylvania in 2004, followed by a Post-baccalaureate program at the State University of New York at Buffalo, School of Medicine and Biomedical Sciences. She went on to complete her Doctorate of Medicine at Albert Einstein College of Medicine, at Yeshiva University in 2011. Heather then completed her residency in obstetrics and gynecology at the National Capital Consortium, Walter Reed National Military Medical Center, and joined the Guthrie Ambulatory Care Center as an attending physician in the department of obstetrics and gynecology in Fort Drum, New York, helping soldiers, their spouses, and veterans. Here, she focused on making sure military women had access to high-quality women's health care during their service.

Dr. Heather Irobunda is certified by the American Board of Obstetrics and Gynecology and licensed by the New York State Board of Medicine, and completed military training in Army Officer Basic Leadership, and Combat Casualty Care. Heather is a Fellow of the American College of Obstetrics and Gynecology. She has also completed two years of medical research, with a primary focus on sexual health.

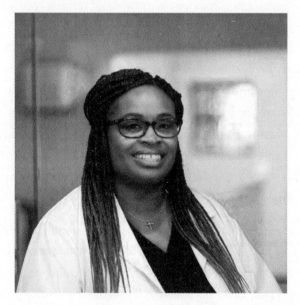

**Dr. Heather Irobunda**

Heather has won a number of awards, most notably the Best Case Report Award from Walter Reed National Military Medical Center in 2013. She has invested her time in teaching and leadership programs, serving as the academics chief resident at the Walter Reed National Military Medical Center, followed by a period of time as the clinical instructor in the physician assistant program at LeMoyne University. Heather shares all she has learned with her online community in order to improve access to reliable, relatable health care information for women.

# A Note from Dr. Heather Irobunda:

After completing four years of medical school, four years of residency, four years as an active-duty Army OB/GYN, and now working in private practice, I've treated *thousands of patients.* This experience has shed light on many themes, but one really stands out to me—there is a *major* gap in access to reliable, transparent online information for women to learn about their health. Having seen both sides of the doctor-patient relationship, I know there are issues with women, particularly women of color, being able to feel comfortable with their health care providers.

I know doctors can be intimidating, but I'm here to show you that they don't have to be. Doctors are patients (and people) too, and I hope to use my experiences, personal and professional, to help all women feel they can make informed decisions and become advocates for themselves. Through my passion for community health paired with my medical expertise, my goal is to help women to feel empowered when seeking medical care.

**In your many years of practice, what is the greatest significant difference that you see when treating Black mothers versus those of other races as it relates to their medical health?**

**Dr. Heather Irobunda:** Black mothers have a unique set of challenges. These challenges are multifactorial. Black mothers have higher rates of health complications in their pregnancies compared to their White counterparts. These health issues include high blood pressure, preeclampsia, and gestational diabetes to name a few. Also, although it is unclear how common mental disorders like depression and anxiety are in the Black community, it is known that Black women are less likely to seek help for these conditions than White women. This difference in accessing mental health care can also have a negative effect on their pregnancies. When looking at psychosocial differences during pregnancy, unfortunately Black women also are more negatively impacted. There are differences in attainment of resources and wealth, and these disparities can negatively impact health, including maternal health.

**What factors in our lifestyle and genetics directly correlate with this difference?**

**DI:** There have also been shown to be increased risks of obesity, high blood pressure, and diabetes in Black women that would cause differences in Black maternal health. Many of these medical issues increase the risk of pregnancy complications. The reasons for these differences are multifactorial. Some of them are due to lack of access to preventative care in communities of color. Also, there are often disparities in access to healthy food in these communities as well. These factors all have an effect on how communities can maintain good health.

Due to institutional racism and other systemic injustices that have had negative impacts on their current socioeconomic status, this can cause Black people to experience stress. The stress can affect pregnancies at alarmingly high rates. Economic stresses, like unemployment and working low wage employment, are also stressors. In medicine, we know that higher levels of stress, depression, and anxiety during pregnancy can also have deleterious effects on growing babies. These can include low birth weight babies and preterm labor. This can also lead to medical and mental health issues in the future for these children, which can affect the next generation of Black people.

There are theories that suggest that, genetically, there are some differences that are shown in Black people, especially Black people in the African diaspora, and an increased risk for certain health issues like high blood pressure. For example, one popular theory is that Black people from the diaspora have higher rates of high blood pressure and that this condition is harder to treat in them due to the Transatlantic slave trade. It is thought that slaves that survived the harsh conditions crossing the Atlantic Ocean survived because they were able to maintain a higher blood pressure which allowed them to withstand the lack of hydration. In this theory it is noted that the genetic makeup of those ancestors has been passed down and now presents itself as high blood pressure in their descendants.

**Let's jump right into the topic of gestational diabetes. What is gestational diabetes and how does it affect Black women more than women of other races?**

**DI:** Gestational diabetes is a condition in which your body does not process sugar in the way that it should, causing your blood sugar to be higher than normal. In order to understand gestational diabetes, it is important to understand how your body handles your blood sugar. There is a hormone called insulin that is created in your pancreas that keeps your blood sugar regulated. Insulin allows your body to store sugar that is circulating in your blood so that you can have enough sugar in your blood when you need it and so that you can save some for later. In nonpregnant people, diabetes mellitus is classified in two ways, type I and type II. Type I is an autoimmune condition in which your body makes antibodies to attack the cells in your pancreas that make insulin causing the body to not be able to put away that insulin, causing the blood sugar to become high. Type II diabetes is when the tissues in your body that normally store sugar because insulin tells them to are more resistant to insulin (as in, they stop listening to insulin so much) and more sugar stays in the blood causing the levels to become high. Gestational diabetes is when this condition, the elevation in blood sugar, occurs during pregnancy. It is believed that this occurs because the placenta releases chemicals during pregnancy that cause the tissue that normally takes in sugar to be more resistant to insulin.

Gestational diabetes can lead to many different poor pregnancy outcomes. Gestational diabetes can cause high-birth-weight babies, large amounts of amniotic fluid (polyhydramnios), preterm delivery, stillbirth, and newborns that require NICU (neonatal intensive care unit) stays. It also makes women 40 to 50 percent more likely to develop diabetes in a nonpregnant state in the future.

Black women are affected by gestational diabetes at an increased rate than their White counterparts. There are many sources of data that have varying numbers for the prevalence of gestational diabetes, but in all of the data, Black women are consistently affected more by gestational diabetes than White women. Other ethnicities, specifically Asian Pacific Islanders and Latinas, also show higher rates than their White counterparts. The increased prevalence of gestational diabetes seems to come from a variety of factors. It appears that being overweight or having a high BMI plays a role in increasing the risk for gestational diabetes, and there is a higher prevalence of obesity in Black women than their White counterparts. Also, diet may contribute to this difference in addition to genetics. There is more research that needs to be done to evaluate these differences.

**How does gestational diabetes correlate to preeclampsia? Can you also define what preeclampsia is and how it affects pregnancy?**

**DI:** Gestational diabetes can increase a woman's risk of developing preeclampsia. The exact way that this happens is not fully known, however there is likely a link with how poorly controlled blood sugar affects your blood vessels. In general, we typically see alterations in the blood vessels in diabetics outside of pregnancy because over time these vessels end up with plaques and injuries to them due to high levels of sugar for long periods of time. In a nonpregnant person, it is what can cause diabetics to have heart attacks, strokes, blindness, and poor circulation, which leads to amputations of limbs. In pregnancy, though, we often do not see these effects because pregnancy (and therefore gestational diabetes) does not last enough time to cause these severe complications. However, we do think that even in the short length of time that a woman has gestational diabetes, it can affect the blood vessels enough to cause preeclampsia.

Preeclampsia is a condition that occurs in pregnancy after twenty weeks. It is a condition that we believe has a vascular origin (although the exact reason is not understood). We do know that it causes a number of symptoms like high blood pressure and high levels of protein in urine. It also can cause vision changes that range from blurry vision to seeing floaters. Other symptoms include abdominal pain that occurs in the right upper part of your abdomen, severe headache, and swelling throughout the body. In severe cases of preeclampsia, it can cause liver and kidney damage, hemorrhage, and even stillbirth. Preeclampsia is a very serious condition and should not be taken lightly, because it could lead to eclampsia in some cases. Eclampsia is when a woman has seizures in addition to some of the aforementioned symptoms. These seizures are scary for a multitude of reasons. First, while a mother is having a seizure, she is not getting a lot of oxygen into her body. This can affect the oxygen that her baby gets through the placenta and can put the baby in danger of brain injuries or stillbirth. Second, these seizures are slightly different from seizures that people with epilepsy can have. These seizures are usually a sign of stroke-like activity in the brain. In other words, the eclamptic seizures can be a sign of stroke activity in the brain that can lead to permanent damage of brain tissue. Both preeclampsia and eclampsia are very scary and severe conditions and some of the biggest concerns that obstetricians have when caring for a pregnant woman.

**Is there a way that doctors test mothers for gestational diabetes? How accurate and necessary is this testing?**

**DI:** There are multiple ways that doctors test mothers for gestational diabetes. Typically, we test all mothers for gestational diabetes between 24 and 28 weeks into pregnancy. The test that we perform for women is called an oral glucose challenge test (GCT). This test lasts one hour and does not require the mother to fast prior to having this lab test done. The mother will come either to the medical office or the lab (however her obstetrician or midwife has it set up) and she will be given a drink. This drink contains fifty grams of glucose. This drink comes in a variety of flavors, but the most common flavor is orange. On a bit of a side note, many women feel that this drink tastes like really sweet, flat, orange soda. After the mother has completed her drink, she waits for one hour and then has her blood drawn. The blood test measures the blood glucose level and shows us how her body reacts and handles glucose (which is sugar). There is no standard cutoff for the blood glucose test because the cutoff values are highly dependent on what region of the United States or even the world that the mother lives in. If the test results show an elevated value over the cutoff, there is further testing necessary. Very rarely does a mother get the diagnosis of gestational diabetes from just this test, because this test just screens for a mother's risk of gestational diabetes. It is not truly meant to diagnose diabetes. If a mother has an elevated value, this shows that she has an elevated risk of having gestational diabetes and she is then required to have further testing to diagnose it. The next test is called an oral glucose tolerance test (GTT). This test is more involved than the GCT. The GTT takes three hours to complete and requires the mother to have a drink with 100g of glucose that is provided by either the laboratory or the medical office. Before the mother has the 100g drink of glucose, she has her blood drawn to see what her fasting glucose level is. After that first blood draw, she drinks the 100g of glucose and then she has her blood drawn once an hour for three hours. After this test is completed, the values are evaluated and if two or more these values are elevated, the mother is diagnosed with gestational diabetes.

Sometimes, an obstetrician will want to test mothers earlier for diabetes. When a woman first goes to see an obstetrician for pregnancy, we will gather a detailed medical history from her. We want to know what her baseline health status is at the start of her pregnancy. We also find out about her family's medical history. Oftentimes, if we encounter women who have family members with diabetes, especially someone closely related to her, like her mother, father, or siblings, this will put her at higher risk for gestational diabetes. Also, if a woman tells us that she has a history of polycystic ovarian syndrome or is overweight or obese, that may also be considered evidence of a higher risk for gestational diabetes. If we find that there is an increased risk of gestational diabetes, we may choose to test a mother earlier in her pregnancy for it. If no diabetes is found during this earlier testing, testing is repeated again at twenty-four to twenty-eight weeks.

**How do diet and exercise play a role in the prevention of gestational diabetes?**

**DI**: Diet and exercise definitely have a role in preventing gestational diabetes. When looking at risk factors for gestational diabetes, higher BMI is one of the risk factors. Also having an elevated hemoglobin A1C. Hemoglobin A1C is a compound we test for in the blood that allows us to see how well your body has been handling sugar. People who suffer from diabetes regularly tend to have an elevation in this value when they are first diagnosed. When they start altering their diet and sometime through the use of medications, they can see this value decrease. There are also people who are prediabetic who have an elevation in this value, but who have not made the threshold of diabetes. Often, when people are prediabetic, it can be reversed with diet and exercise. So using this same logic, improving or maintaining a healthy, well-balanced diet and including cardiovascular exercise can reduce your risk of developing gestational diabetes.

**In your medical opinion, do you believe that it is safe for pregnant women that have not exercised before pregnancy to start during pregnancy?**

**DI**: It is definitely safe to start exercising during pregnancy! In April 2020, the American College of Obstetricians and Gynecologists wrote a committee opinion on this very topic. Many women may be concerned about the health of their baby or about risking pregnancy complications by starting an exercise routine, however research shows that women who exercise in pregnancy have lower risks of gestational diabetes, preeclampsia, and Cesarean delivery. Most women who get pregnant would be considered healthy enough to begin an exercise routine before they get pregnant, and fortunately, pregnancy does not change that in many of those women.

Usually, we do recommend refraining from starting very intense forms of exercise if you had not been doing them before. Examples of intense forms of exercise would be marathon training and extreme bodybuilding. However, the recommendation from the Department of Health and Human Services and the American Academy of Cardiology is to participate in at least 150 minutes of cardiovascular exercise per week. If a woman has any concerns about starting up a new exercise routine, do not hesitate to see your obstetric provider to address them.

**What are some ways that women who are planning to get pregnant but have a history of diabetes in their family can prepare for pregnancy?**

**DI:** One of the most important ways for women who are planning to get pregnant to prepare for pregnancy is to visit their gynecologist and have a discussion with them about your plans. This allows for an open dialogue about your health and your family health history. Establishing this relationship allows your gynecologist to do any necessary tests to see if you may already have diabetes or signs of prediabetes. It may also allow them to do other testing in general to make sure that your overall health is good. In addition, you and your gynecologist can discuss your current exercise habits and diet and make sure they are in the best place before you get pregnant.

**It was important to include a full breakdown on gestational diabetes in this book, not as a way to induce fear but to make mothers aware. Do you have any words of encouragement for mothers that may experience gestational diabetes during their pregnancy?**

**DI:** We are here for you. And by "we," I mean your obstetricians! Getting a diagnosis of gestational diabetes can be so scary. Especially when you find out all of the negative ways it can impact your pregnancy. However, there is a lot of information that we know about gestational diabetes that allows us to help you through your pregnancy better. Many times, we as humans think of the worst-case scenario. We may look at all of the possibilities for a negative outcome and believe that it will happen to us. Most times those negative outcomes will not happen to us. Staying proactive and advocating for the health of yourself and your growing baby will help minimize the worst-case scenarios in most women. Staying positive has a wonderful effect on your body, especially when dealing with a medical problem like gestational diabetes. It decreases stress hormones that can worsen medical problems, and it can make you work harder to stay on top of healthy habits that can reduce the effect that gestational diabetes will have on your pregnancy.

*Thank you to Dr. Heather Irobunda for her insight on this very important conversation. If you are experiencing any complications due to pregnancy, please speak with your medical provider. To learn more about Dr. Irobunda or to inquire about medical services, visit IrobundaMD.com.*

## Chapter Three

# All Jokes Aside, Speak Up, Sis: What You Need to Know about Black Maternal Health

*Sometimes, I feel discriminated against, but it does not make me angry. It merely astonishes me. How can any deny themselves the pleasure of my company? It's beyond me.*

—Zora Neale Hurston

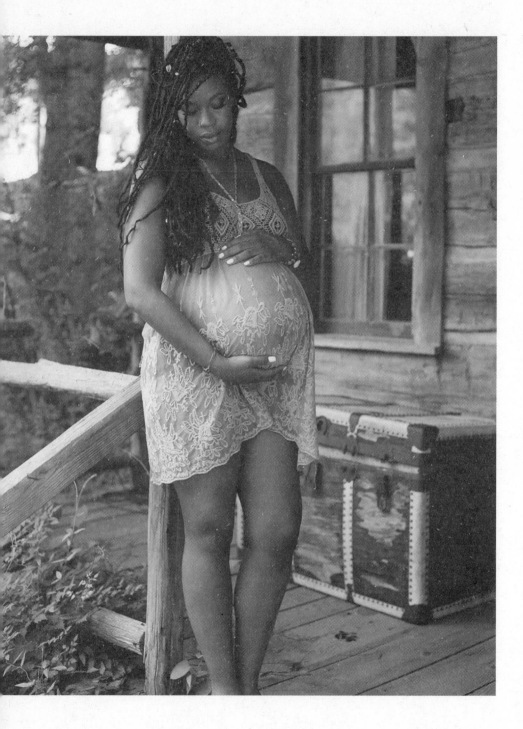

Earlier in the book, I gave insight on the importance of the *Black Moms Blog* and why I created it. When I was pregnant with my daughter, I searched online for information on pregnancy and childbirth from a woman like me—young, Black, and millennial. Finding pregnancy information was not impossible. There were books, apps, and websites like What to Expect and the Mayo Clinic. I found social media accounts from blonde women living in three-story homes with perfectly clean kitchens and fantastic husbands who brought them breakfast in bed. Their children were manicured and neat, smiling from ear to ear. The few Black mom bloggers I found kept up the same aesthetic. Everything there was the same as with the White mom, only their skin color was different.

I could not find articles that dug a little deeper into the Black experience of parenting or spoke in a way that I felt that I could really relate to. I wanted to read articles that noted key cultural references and made me laugh. I know what it is like to have my ears burned by a straightening comb on Sunday mornings, I needed that. I wanted to read about the experiences of Black women who could relate to having to go get a switch off a tree and how we were steadfast about raising our children differently. Keep in mind, this was nearly a decade ago. Thankfully, now we can open our social media apps and find moms that look like us and speak our language. Mothers who are first-generation anything in their families: first-generation breast feeders, first-generation natural birthers, degreed Black women, Black women raising their children in two-parent households and Black women who are truly unapologetic. You will find a wide array of Black mothers that focus on natural hair, birth options, single parenting, coparenting, marriage life, and so much more.

The parenthood industry has finally begun to include us in its narrative. Companies started spending money with Black mom bloggers because they knew that we had options. Why would I shop with a baby brand that never featured one sister of color in their marketing campaigns when I had Sis over here selling organic belly butter and baby cloth wraps straight from the motherland? I am beyond grateful for this evolution. It has led to many opportunities for mothers to gain insight from women that look like them—which is hopefully why you are reading this book. You know the importance of having someone in your corner who truly knows your experience. It is crucial that we discuss real-life situations that you may experience during your prenatal appointments.

Being a mom can feel overwhelming. You are going to find yourself at the center of all sorts of advice being thrown your way. If this is your first baby, it may all seem alarming in the beginning, but stay strong, Sis, you got this. As I look back on my experience with pregnancy, one of the most intimidating experiences was going to my prenatal appointments. When I found out I was pregnant, I did not have health insurance. I had to sign up for Medicaid which meant I had limited options in which doctors I could see and the care that would be provided to me. It meant that as soon as I walked into the doctor's office, I was judged. I was young, single (because I was not married), and Black. I was a walking, twenty-two-year-old statistic. Even though my daughter's father attended every doctor's visit with me, and we were well dressed, polite, and on time, it did not stop the judgmental statements and lack of care from our doctor. Every doctor I saw thought she was my mama because clearly a girl like me had none.

It is necessary that you be prepared for this if you find yourself in this situation. It is not just important during your prenatal appointments but also during your child's birth. If you are too afraid to express your concerns, you will find yourself unable to say when a certain jolt feels painful or you feel unusually exhausted.

# We Are More Than a Statistic

Black women are statistically more likely to receive subpar medical care and suffer from poorer health outcomes. Consequently, this leads to higher death rates related to pregnancy and childbirth. Compared to White women, Black women are two to six times more likely to die during childbirth.[1] The Black maternal mortality rate does not care if you are rich or poor. Powerful women like Serena Williams and Beyoncé have spoken openly about complications and treatments they experienced during childbirth. While there is not any clear explanation for why Black women die at a higher rate than their counterparts, many researchers have cited institutional racism, sexism, and, at times, financial barriers as leading factors.

When a Black woman expresses discomfort, her words can be considered more of a rudimentary complaint than an actual concern. Colorism can also play a major role in this. Darker women are seen as more strong and tough, whereas our lighter counterparts may seem more helpless and tender. This is not to put dark and light at opposing ends of the spectrum. As a Black woman, regardless of your complexion, you still face a higher likelihood of receiving subpar treatment while pregnant. It is

1    www.ncbi.nlm.nih.gov/pmc/articles/PMC1595019/

important to speak up. If you are able to, find a provider that understands your complications as a Black mother. Ask deep questions about their statistics as a birth doctor. Do not be afraid to ask the hard questions.

- Has your health care provider heard of Black maternal health?

- Does your health care provider take additional precautions to make sure they are actively listening to the concerns of their patients? (Active listening looks like undivided attention, direct eye contact, taking notes when you express concerns, and answering your questions without making you feel rushed or silly for asking them.)

- Do you feel comfortable using your voice openly with your health care provider?

- What are their statistics in caring for Black patients?

- What sort of aftercare does your health care provider offer for mothers once birth has commenced?

# Find a Proper Advocate

Having a proper advocate during your pregnancy and birthing process can be a matter of life and death. Even if you feel up to speed during your pregnancy, you can still find yourself unable to properly advocate for your needs during birth. While your doctor hopefully respects your wishes, you will indeed be in a more vulnerable position during labor. Thankfully, you have many options when it comes to finding birth workers, and with social media it has become easier to find a birth worker that looks like you. Later in the book we will talk about your options for where and how to birth, but for now let's focus on your options for advocacy.

**Please note, I am not a medical professional and cannot give medical advice on pregnancy or advocacy.**

# Your Partner

When I became pregnant at twenty-two years old, I was completely unaware of my options for a birth advocate. For me, my partner was the best solution. While we did not do a shabby job in getting our daughter into the world, looking back, I would have hired a birth worker.

If you choose to have your partner as your birth advocate, it is important to include them on your birth plan, evaluating what your options are in a critical situation, and making sure they can properly communicate with the hospital staff during your labor. Your partner should be comfortable advocating for your rights while seeing you in pain. Your partner will benefit from learning how to comfort you through pain while also upholding your desire to have a med-free birth, an epidural, or any other intervention.

It can be a lot of pressure on your partner to show up and be all of these things for you though. Sometimes, your partner just needs to be your support, and a birth worker can be the person to advocate for you. Your partner can hold your hand. If you do not have a partner, call your best friend.

# Birth Doula

According to the American Pregnancy Association, a doula is a professional trained in childbirth who provides emotional, physical, and educational support to a mother who is expecting, is experiencing labor, or has recently given birth. Doulas can be extremely essential during the pregnancy, birth, and afterbirth experience. While doulas are not medically trained, they work to act more as your pregnancy and birth coach and advocate during childbirth.

Earlier, we covered a few reasons why your partner may or may not be the best advocate for you. A doula is trained specifically in these areas to help communicate your needs to your OB (obstetrician) or midwife during the birthing process. Statistics show that women who hire a doula during pregnancy are the least likely to need a Cesarean birth and tend to stick to their desire, if intended, to have a natural birthing process. Doulas are sort of like your knowledgeable pregnant best friend. You can discuss birthing techniques, ask all the questions you are slightly freaking out about, and even ask for an occasional belly rub or two. When it comes time for labor, they will be the support system reminding you to breathe while at the same time making sure your delivering doctor or midwife is keeping your needs first. Thanks to sources like BlackDoulas.org, you can find a doula of color in your area that will keep your needs first. While doulas are not normally covered in your health insurance, their services are reasonably priced, with most charging between $800 and $2,500 per client.

# Midwife

According to WebMD, a midwife is a trained health professional who helps healthy women during labor, delivery, and after the birth of their babies. A midwife can legally birth your babies at home, in a hospital, or at a birthing center. Midwives typically only work with healthy pregnancies, but if a pregnancy is considered high risk or consists of multiple babies, your midwife can shadow your doctor. If you are pregnant with multiples, you can still hire a midwife, but most doctors suggest still going to your OB because a birth of multiples can be more complicated.

There are three common types of midwives:

- Certified Nurse Midwife (CNM): A CNM is an RN, or Registered Nurse, who has completed training and graduated from a national accredited nurse-midwifery program. A person with this title can deliver babies in all fifty states.

- Certified Midwife (CM): A CM does not have the accreditation as a nurse but has a bachelor's or master's degree in a health field and has successfully passed an accredited midwifery national education program. A CM is only permitted to deliver babies in a handful of states.

- Certified Professional Midwife (CPM): A CPM is also a non-nurse midwife that has passed a national exam. This exam does not have to be at an accredited institution. A CPM does have training and clinical experience in childbirth in and out of the hospital. CPMs are not permitted to practice in all states.

Your midwife is kind of like your supremely educated pregnant bestie that can provide more medical advice and actually birth your baby at the same time. You can ask your midwife the same sort of questions you can ask your doula, but a midwife can also:

- Deliver your baby
- Admit and discharge you from the hospital
- Do prenatal exams and order tests
- Make doctor referrals
- Monitor your physical and psychological health
- Provide family planning and preconception care[2]

Midwives are typically covered in most insurance plans as long as your baby is birthed in a hospital or birthing center. Insurance does not normally cover midwives for home births. The average cost of a midwife is around $3,500, but if applicable, your insurance will cover a partial or total amount of their fees.

# Create a Birth Plan

Creating a birth plan can also help to get your partner, your OB or midwife, and your doula all on the same page. No one has time to explain over and over how you want your birth to go, especially when you are already in labor. A birth plan is a game plan for your labor and delivery. It should include some important details about how your room should look, your pain medicine preferences, a safe word (my own personal addition to the normal list of things you should include in a birth plan), and your aftercare newborn instructions. With apps and websites like Canva, you can create a

2    www.webmd.com/baby/what-is-a-midwife-twins.

fun and colorful birth plan for your loved ones and medical staff. Along with creating your birth plan, I would also suggest creating a musical playlist of your favorite songs that you visualize getting you through your labor. I would recommend mixing it up from Sade to Beyoncé to 2 Chainz. You are going to need a bit of serene, girl power, and ratchet all grouped into one.

# Sample Birth Plan

Name: _____ Due Date: _____

## Attendees At Birth

Partner: _____

Friends: _____

Family: _____

Birth Worker: _____

Children: _____

## Labor (Circle which applies)

Birthing Stool    Birthing Chair    Squatting Bar    Birthing Pool/Tub

Let my water break on its own.                    YES            NO

I would like light food during labor             YES            NO

Fetal Monitoring:    Continuous    Intermittent    Wireless for Movement

## Pain Management (Circle which applies)

Acupressure    Bath/Shower    Breathing Techniques/Distraction

Hot/Cold Therapy    Hypnobirthing    Massage

## Medication

I would like pain medication offered to me.      YES            NO

I will ask for pain medication.                  YES            NO

If I decide I want medicinal pain relief, I'd prefer: _____

Epidural is okay.                                YES            NO

Systemic medication.                             YES            NO

I would like Pitocin if labor stalls.            YES            NO

## Comfort

| | | |
|---|---|---|
| I will provide my own music. | YES | NO |
| I would like the lights dimmed. | YES | NO |
| I will labor in my own clothing. | YES | NO |
| Photo/video is allowed. | YES | NO |

## Birth

| | | |
|---|---|---|
| I will push on instinct. | YES | NO |
| I would like to be coached on when to push and for how long. | YES | NO |

### I would like to birth in these positions: (Circle which applies)

Semi-reclining    Squatting    Side-lying position

Hands and Knees    Whatever feels right at the time

## Vaginal Birth

| | | |
|---|---|---|
| Please provide a mirror so I can see my birth. | YES | NO |
| I would like to touch my baby's head during crowning. | YES | NO |
| I would like to give birth without an episiotomy. | YES | NO |
| I want my partner to catch our baby. | YES | NO |

## C-Section

In case of a C-section:

Who is allowed in the room: _____

| | | |
|---|---|---|
| I would like to see my baby delivered. | YES | NO |
| I would like immediate skin-to-skin contact. | YES | NO |

## Postpartum

| | | |
|---|---|---|
| I would like immediate skin-to-skin contact. | YES | NO |
| I would like a lotus birth. | YES | NO |
| I would like my partner to cut the umbillical cord. | YES | NO |
| I would like to delay my baby's bath. | YES | NO |

| | | |
|---|---|---|
| I would like to breastfeed exclusively. | YES | NO |
| I would like to breastfeed and formula feed. | YES | NO |
| I would like to use formula provided by the hospital. | YES | NO |
| I will provide my own formula. | YES | NO |
| I would like my baby to have a pacifier. | YES | NO |
| Do not offer my baby sugar water. | YES | NO |
| I would like to keep my placenta. | YES | NO |
| All newborn procedures must be done with my partner present. | YES | NO |
| All newborn procedures must be done in my presence. | YES | NO |

The baby cannot be taken from the room without either of these people present:

_____

| | | |
|---|---|---|
| The baby should be roomed with me twenty-four hours a day while in the hospital. | YES | NO |
| The baby should only be roomed with me while I am awake. | YES | NO |
| I would like my baby to be vaccinated. | YES | NO |

## Cord Blood (Circle which applies)

| Donate to a public bank | Donate to a private bank | Neither |
|---|---|---|

## Circumcision

| | | |
|---|---|---|
| I want him circumcised at the hospital. | YES | NO |
| I will delay circumcision. | YES | NO |
| I don't want him circumcised. | YES | NO |

# Your Room

This section of your birth plan will depend on a few things. If you are birthing at home or in a birth center (we will discuss these choices later on), you will have a little more flexibility in how you want your room to look. You can add in candles, essential oils, herbs, and music. Dimmed lights are important too. Hospital births may not allow candles, but you may be able to bring an essential oil diffuser. Check with your hospital to find out your specific regulations.

## Who Do You Want in the Room

We need an entire chapter for this. Stay tuned, Sis.

# Pain Management

How do you plan to manage your pain? If you are having a vaginal birth, you will need to decide between a natural birth and a medicated birth. A natural birth, which can include a water birth, means that you do not plan on using any pain medication to birth your baby. This may also vary if your medical provider decides to induce your birth with Pitocin. Pitocin is a form of oxytocin administered by IV which can be used to start your labor, speed up labor, or can be given after birth to control blood flow. Pitocin is normally used when you have passed the standard forty-one-week mark in pregnancy or your baby is lacking in fluids. Because Pitocin can be used to induce and speed up labor, it can also cause more intense labor cramps. Talk to your medical provider about your options with Pitocin so that you are properly informed before labor begins.

If you choose to have a medicated birth, your medical provider will most likely give you an epidural. An epidural is an anesthetic that blocks pain to a specific part of the body. Receiving an epidural does not take away feeling. Instead, it numbs your nerve impulses from your lower spinal area. Epidurals are effective at relieving pain caused during labor and delivery.

Listen, Mama, whichever route you choose, pain-free or medicated, the most important part of labor is birthing a healthy baby and healing a healthy mom. Do not feel guilty for any decision you make. It is yours.

# Aftercare

Your birth plan should include an aftercare section for you and your baby. Do you have specific needs after birth? This should include matters like who cuts the cord or whether you would you prefer for a lotus birth (a lotus birth is where you leave the cord attached after birth), breastfeeding or bottle feeding, whether you want your baby bathed after being born, and if you are having a boy, whether he should be circumcised. Do not forget about yourself. If you want to take the perfect "Mommy and Me" birth photo, you may want to include that no photos should be taken until you give the okay. Also, let those in the room know ahead of time to please not post reveal photos of your newborn until you are able to post your own.

By properly preparing for your impending birth, you will greatly reduce the chances of any mishaps that could happen during labor. Remember this: Speak up for yourself. Advocate for yourself. Have someone else advocate for you.

# Options for Pregnant Women during COVID-19...or Any Other Global Pandemic

It would be remiss of me not to include a portion of this guidebook relating to our reality. We are currently in a global pandemic as I write this. Our world has been turned upside down due to COVID-19, which has caused each and every person around the globe to find a new normal. COVID is not discriminatory. It does not care if you are Black or White, young or old, although statistically more Black people have been affected. All people are susceptible to catching the virus. Those with compromised immune systems are more at risk and so are pregnant women. While the pandemic will eventually come to an end as all things do, it has made us more aware of what we can do during these trying times. I realize that our pregnant mamas are in for a different type of battle. With the hospitals being filled to capacity and the fear of catching this debilitating virus, many are left wondering, "What are my options when it comes to my birth?"

## Should I Still Give Birth in a Hospital?

Hospital births are under major stress. Mothers are being dressed in full hazmat suits before entering hospitals. Husbands and support systems are not being allowed to attend the birth of their babies. Needless to say, no mom has been properly prepared to give birth under these circumstances.

In conversation with Latham Thomas, founder of Mama Glow, we discussed what options mothers have as it pertains to a hospital birth. Latham's number one suggestion? Hire a doula. No matter where you are in your pregnancy, it is not too late to have a doula coach you through your birth. Latham says, as a doula, one of her goals is to help control the narrative for a birth mama. Instead of focusing on what is going wrong right now, a doula helps a mama learn how to breathe, control her stress, be her own advocate, and deliver a healthy newborn. Even though your doula may not be able to attend your birth due to the pandemic and hospitals putting restrictions on how many people are allowed in a birthing room, they can join you as a virtual doula and coach you over the phone or computer.

# Remember to Mind Your Health and Stay Calm

Whether it be COVID-19 or a future pandemic, always remember that your health and the health of your baby are of utmost importance. Make sure you are getting plenty of rest and eating well, and practice social distancing from others who are sick or could become sick. There has not been much medical information released on how COVID can affect your pregnancy or your breastfeeding, but hopefully in the future we will know more. No matter what side you are on when it comes to the severity of COVID-19, understand that as a pregnant woman, compromising your immune system is not a risk worth taking. Wait it out, Sis. Don't attend the party if you can help it. Send someone else to the store. We are aiming for healthy pregnancies with peace of mind.

## Chapter Four

# A Conversation with Tracie Collins, Founder of the National Black Doulas Association

*If you prioritize yourself,*
*you are going to save yourself.*

—Gabrielle Union

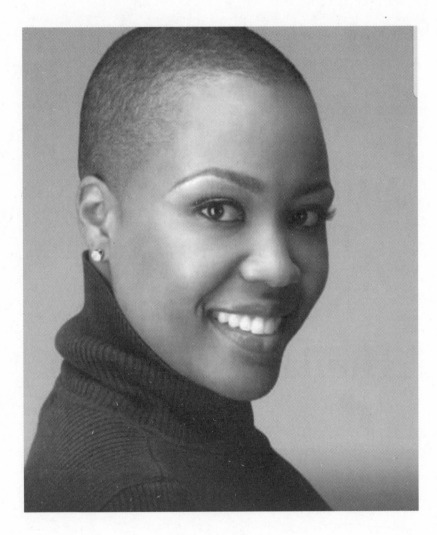

**In the last chapter, we** took an in-depth look into the steps you can take to ensure your voice is respected during your pregnancy and labor experience. Selecting an advocate will be a very important part of your pregnancy. You want to choose a professional who makes you feel heard and who honors your voice. Tracie Collins, founder of the National Black Doulas Association joins us for an interview to explain why she decided to become a doula, her passion for Black motherhood, and to provide us with pertinent questions so that you can be equipped to interview your own birth advocate.

Tracie began her career in the birth doula field in 2000 after her second child was born. She has attended over 1,500 births, with families birthing in hospitals, birth centers, and at homes throughout the San Francisco Bay area and beyond. In 2002, Tracie completed the Elizabeth Davis' Heart & Hands Midwifery Incentives Program. Upon completion, she was the only student from that class to be selected as an apprentice midwife for Sacred Body Midwifery in San Francisco. After her apprenticeship, she worked as a midwife with Sacred Grove Midwifery alongside Asatu Hall.

Due to her vast experience and educational background, Tracie has developed a method to help prepare the mother's body for more efficient labor through proper prenatal nutrition and more. She has combined the approach with laboring positions, techniques, and her extensive knowledge of and foundation in midwifery, applying each to the birth process in such a way that doctors, nurses, and other birthing professionals trust and seek out her expertise. Tracie is greatly in demand and comes with an extremely high level of regard, experience, and longevity in the birthing field. She has worked for over two decades in many settings to empower and provide expectant families with the best support possible.

In 2017 Tracie founded the National Black Doulas Association, which has quickly become the leading resource for Black birthing professionals to be found by birthing families. The NBDA has a special emphasis on educational and economic development for birthing professionals, all while standing on the birth principles of midwifery.

# An Interview with Tracie Collins

**What made you become a doula that specifically focuses on Black motherhood?**

Tracie Collins: When I became a doula in 2000, I was on my path toward becoming a CPM (certified professional midwife). It wasn't until 2017 that I founded the NBDA (National Black Doulas Association), with a primary focus on doing my part to connect more Black birthing families with Black doulas to help fight the Black maternal death rate in this country.

**What is the role of a doula during pregnancy and childbirth, and how does that differ from the role of a midwife?**

TC: The simplest way to describe it is the midwife does everything medical. The doula's role is nonmedical. The doula is there to provide informational, emotional, and physical support to the prenatal, birthing and postpartum family. The doula, once they are hired by the expectant family, meets with the family during their gestational period to help prepare them for the birthing process. The doula involves the birthing partner as well because this is their birth too. The doula helps to empower the family through information and education. Your doula also helps to provide understanding of procedures and policies the birthing family may face during the course of labor and delivery. The doula teaches and provides various comfort measures throughout the course of labor and delivery, supports breastfeeding, and so much more. The doula has a deep understanding of the physiology of labor, what is happening at every stage, to help guide the process and be the gatekeeper of safety. A good doula also understands the professional hierarchy within hospitals, to get results if need be.

**As a doula, what is your overall mission when working with mothers?**

**TC:** Doulas work with birthing people. More than just women are birthing, and we have to recognize that. All families are deserving of support. The doula's overall mission is: "Healthy birthing person, healthy baby, and whatever we need to do to get there." Oftentimes that means veering from the birthing parents' wishes or preferences because doulas are navigators of safety.

**What is one of the biggest myths you have heard about doulas and how have you worked in your career to counteract that?**

**TC:** One of the biggest myths is that doulas are glorified labor coaches, and any person can do this work, like a family member or friend. This is simply incorrect. A doula is a highly trained professional with an area of expertise or focus. Doulas are trained to identify potential issues during pregnancy, labor, and postpartum that oftentimes get dismissed or overlooked in the medical system. Doulas work in conjunction with the medical staff to support, not to overstep or undermine, the licensed medical team of professionals. Truth be told, a really good doula will see potential issues that medicine can miss or choose to ignore, especially if the birthing person is a person of color. They will then introduce techniques and processes to ensure the health of the birthing person and baby.

**What are questions that you think a pregnant mother should consider asking when looking for a doula?**

**TC:** Here is a list of potential questions on the National Black Doulas Association site that myself and many of the NBDA members came up with. These are questions that you can ask when interviewing for your own doula.

## QUESTIONS FOR BIRTH DOULAS

◊ **How many clients do you take per month?**

Industry standard is three to six clients per month. Doulas are used to juggling clients and due dates. An EDD is just an estimated date of delivery, not a guarantee. Doulas focus on months, not dates. Anywhere between thirty-seven and forty-two weeks is considered full term.

◊ **What is your stance on medicated vs. unmedicated birth?**

◊ **Do you have a particular coaching style?**

◊ **How many prenatal visits do you offer and what is covered in each visit? Postpartum visits?**

Doulas offer between two and three prenatal visits. However, some may offer more or less depending on circumstance and need.

◇ **How are payments structured? Do you require a portion down? Full payment up front? Payment plans?**

This will differ per Doula.

◇ **Do you accept FSA or HSA payments?**

◇ **Do you have a time limit on support?**

There may be a clause in the contract that states that after a certain amount of hours a doula reserves the right to call another doula to support for long births extending over twelve hours or more.

◇ **What is your backup doula policy?**

All doulas should have a backup policy in the event she is at another birth or sick. Remember, life happens!

◇ **How do you support, educate, and help involve my partner?**

It is your partner's birth too! Partners experience birth on so many levels that deserve respect and honor. How the doula involves the birth partner in the entire process from beginning to end is very important to know.

◇ **Do you have an "on call" policy?**

Some doulas only go "on call" for your birth at a certain number of weeks' gestation. This is very important to know in the event of a preterm labor and delivery.

◊ **What happens if I end up needing a C-section? Will I get a partial refund?**

◊ **Do you have any specialties that can aid in my overall birth experience? Is there any extra fee?**

Doulas can also be massage therapists, acupuncturists, chefs, Ayurvedic practitioners, placenta practitioners, belly binders, and so much more. What other skills, if any, will she have to offer throughout your course of care with them as your doula?

◊ **Have you supported many women of color delivering in a hospital setting?**

This is good to know when it comes to hospital culture, policy, and procedures for dealing with women of color, especially Black women within the confines of Western medicine. Are they being heard? Are their wishes being respected?

◊ **What if I need to be induced? How does your support change, if at all?**

Medical inductions can change the trajectory of labor. Does a doula offer support and is she familiar with the induction procedures at the local hospitals? Can she provide education in that regard?

◊ **Have you supported women of size?**

There are biases in Western medicine when it comes to women being plus size. This can impact the level of care they receive greatly. Does the doula have experience in supporting the birthing parent when facing such discrimination?

◇ **What is your experience in working with the LGBTQIA community?**

Does the doula have experience in supporting all family structures? Are there any biases or prejudices present? Does the doula have experience in advocating for this community within hospital settings? If so, ask for an example.

◇ **What has been your experience in supporting a transgender birthing parent?**

◇ **What is your experience in lactation support?**

If the doula isn't a CLC (Certified Lactation Counselor) or IBCLC (International Board-Certified Lactation Consultant), does she have access to resources that offer home visits? It's best to identify one before going into labor. Remember, the lactation consultant is a part of the birthing team.

◇ **Have you ever supported solo parents?**

There are many parents who have chosen to birth solo or whose life circumstances have led them there. What does the doula support look like in that case? How extended is your community?

◇ **How long have you been in this field? Are you affiliated with any organizations we can reference?**

The length of time one has been in this field is not the sole indicator of a good doula. However, are they supported by or are they a part of any reputable organizations that are nationally recognized? This is another valuable way of looking at this.

◇ **Have you had experience working with VBAC (vaginal birth after cesarean) moms?**

◊ Do you have a birth that sticks out in your memory that you feel you learned the most from?

◊ How has this experience shaped you as a doula?

◊ How do you work with the hospital staff or birthing team?

◊ What is your timeframe for our decision?

As stated above, one to two weeks is customary. However, the doula may have another policy in place for her practice.

## QUESTIONS FOR POSTPARTUM DOULAS

◊ Are you certified/trained?

If so, by which organization?

◊ Do you have current infant/adult CPR training?

◊ Do you have a copy of your most recent certification?

◊ What is your availability? Days, evenings, overnights, weekends, etc.?

◊ Does your rate adjust with that? If so, by how much?

◊ What is your fee? What services does this fee cover?

◊ Do we have to book a minimum number of hours to lock in services?

◊ Are there any additional services you offer? (For example: placenta encapsulation, belly wrapping, etc.)

◊ Do you have a criminal background check?

◊ Do you have references I can contact or reviews I can read?

◊ Do you have experience supporting families with twins, triplets, or a special-needs newborn?

◊ Do you have a backup doula just in case of emergencies or conflicts in scheduling?

◊ Are your vaccinations current, such as the flu shot or whooping cough?

◊ Does your service cover errands? (Just in case of C-section)

◊ Do you offer any other skills that we should know about that would be relevant?

## QUESTIONS FOR SPECIALIZED DOULAS

There are doulas that specialize in areas outside of birth and postpartum. These doulas are trained and support women and families going through miscarriage, abortion, and even death. Here are just a few questions to ask to help guide this delicate time in one's life.

◊ What led you to this field?

Doulas have all kinds of reasons, sometimes personal, that have led them to this specific field. Asking this question is a great way of learning if there are some relatable experiences there.

◊ What has been the most beneficial aspect to you in doing this kind of work?

◊ Have there been circumstances that were too hard for you to support?

◊ What is the timeframe for working with you?

Depending upon need, support may vary.

◊ **Do you have other resources that would be beneficial for me during this time?**

Local services that will aid in the healing and transition process during this time.

◊ **How do you support immediate family, if any, affected by this situation?**

This can apply to a hospice situation for death doulas, as well as those offering sibling support in the event of miscarriage.

**Why is hiring a doula important for a pregnant Black mother, specifically?**

**TC:** Hiring a doula is imperative for a Black birthing person because they want to live through the birthing process, period! Delivering a baby in American hospitals has proven time and time again not to be safe for Black people. To understand birthing in America today, you must first understand the history of birth in this country as it pertains to Black people. Our bodies have been raped, experimented on, ignored, abused, and mutilated by the very institutions we've been taught to trust. Enough of that. It is time that Black people and POC reclaim what has been stolen and reclaim our full autonomy over ourselves. One must do that through education and not by trusting the "white coat" with our most prized possessions, ourselves!

**What advice would you give to a woman preparing for motherhood?**

**TC:** #DeepSigh. There really is no true preparation for parenthood. First I would say, do a real self-analysis: are you emotionally, financially, mentally, and spiritually ready? Do you have a community of support? (Because it takes a village, seriously!) Be vulnerable enough to ask for help every step of the way. There is strength in vulnerability.

If you desire to have or already have a birth partner—I say "if" because that is a personal decision, and one may desire to be a solo parent if they choose—make sure your relationship is healthy and strong enough to go the next level into parenthood. You should ask yourself what values are important to you that you want to pass down to your child(ren). What will be your legacy? What generational curses will you be breaking? Make sure you save money! Have good insurance: medical, life, and otherwise.

Determine how you feel about vaccinations and look into your state regulations in regard to vaccines and the educational system's requirements for attending school. Ask yourself the hard questions, like how you plan on educating your child. Home, public, or private school?

*To learn more about Tracie Collins or NBDA, you can visit their website at BlackDoulas.org.*

# A Quick Peek into the "Vaccination Conversation"

Vaccinations are a controversial topic for parents. Each family should feel comfortable choosing what is best for their family and their children when it comes to immunizations. Let's go over the basics of what vaccinations are and how they relate to your pregnancy.

Vaccinations are administered by an injection into the body as a primary means of preventing certain pathogens that can result in serious illness or death. The vaccination familiarizes the body with the pathogen and trains the immune system to recognize it and to eliminate it if you should ever get sick. The premise of vaccinations is that, through herd immunity, the vaccination prevents widespread illness. Herd immunity is when the majority of people become vaccinated or immune to a certain disease, preventing the spread to others.

Vaccinations over the years have proved quite a sensitive topic for discussion. Vaccinations can have common side effects for infants that include soreness at the injection site, fussiness, exhaustion, and a low-grade fever. Each family should do proper research to decide what the best decision for their family and babies is when it comes to vaccinations.

You should make decisions regarding vaccinations while you are pregnant. Your medical advocate will most likely ask whether or not you are planning to vaccinate your baby, if you are choosing certain vaccinations and not others, or delaying the vaccination schedule. The vaccination schedule begins at birth and continues on throughout your lifetime. Here is a basic schedule chart on the vaccination timeline created by Healthline.com.

| Name of Vaccine | Age | How many shots? |
| --- | --- | --- |
| Hepatitis B | Birth | A second at 1–2 months, a third at 6–18 months |
| Rotavirus (RV) | 2 months | A second at 4 months, a third at 6 months |
| Diphtheria, tetanus, and whooping cough (DTaP) | 2 months | A second at 4 months, a third at 6 months, a fourth at 16–18 months; then every 10 years |
| Haemophilus influenzae type b (Hib) | 2 months | A second at 4 months, a third at 6 months, a fourth at 12–15 months |
| Pneumococcal conjugate vaccine PCV13 | 2 months | A second at 4 months, a third at 6 months, a fourth between months 12 and 15 |
| Inactivated Polio Vaccine (IPV) | 2 months | A second at 4 months, a third at 6–18 months, a fourth at 4 to 6 years |
| Influenza | 6 months | Repeat yearly |
| Measles, mumps, and rubella (MMR) | 12–15 months | A second at 4–6 years |
| Varicella | 12–15 months | A second at 4–6 years |
| Hepatitis A | 12–23 months | A second at 6 months after the first |

| Human papillomavirus (HPV) | 11–12 years old | 2-shot series 6 months apart |
| --- | --- | --- |
| Meningococcal conjugate (MenACWY) | 11–12 years old | Booster at 16 years old |
| serogroup B meningococcal (MenB) | 16–18 years old | |
| Pneumococcal (PPSV23) | 19–65+ years old | |
| Herpes zoster (Shingles—RZV formulation) | two doses at 50 years old | |

Pregnancy can be very intense, but the more knowledgeable you are the more prepared you can feel passing this major life milestone. Pregnancy is not all about the medical lingo and doctors though. The very fun parts of pregnancy include being able to wear adorable maternity clothes, decorating your baby's room, and finally becoming a part of the coveted "mom's club" we see in the world of social media. Before we jump into that, have you even considered how you plan to announce your pregnancy? Let's go over the dos and don'ts in the next chapter.

## Chapter Five

# Announcing Your Pregnancy in the Age of Social Media

*The term "late bloomer" implies that we're all supposed to bloom at the same time and that's just not true...or that you can't "bloom" more than once. We will live through multiple versions of ourselves during our time here.*

—Myleik Teele

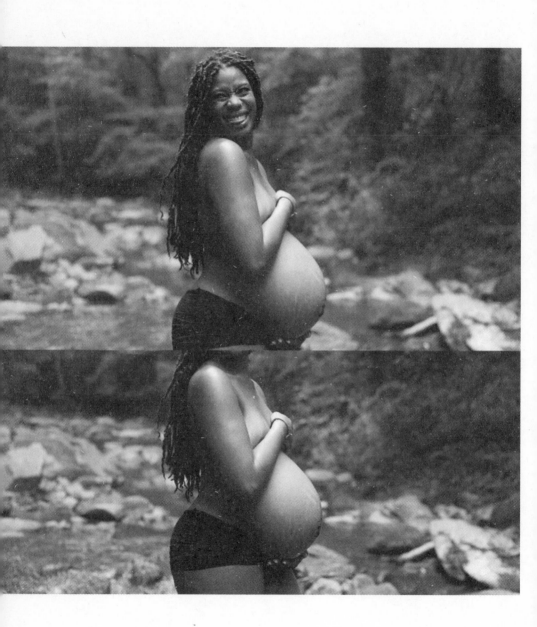

**There used to be a** simpler time in the world when you only had three ways of communicating: 1) Face to face, 2) by rotary telephone, and 3) by mail. Your only concern was the people in the city or town in which you lived and a few distant relatives you only had to see over holiday break. This was the perfect time to make uncomfortable declarations—like when my mother announced to my entire family that I had started my period over Thanksgiving dinner at my grandma's house. I was twelve.

In this day and age, we have more than a dozen ways of communicating, and because of cell phones we are always expected to be responsive immediately. Gone are the times of calling someone's house, leaving a message on their answering machine, and having to wait for them to call back once they are home. Our anxiety levels were lower. We were more patient. The stress of telling those we love about our impending baby bump stayed a family affair instead of becoming a worldwide announcement.

I imagine that back in the day a woman would just show up at her grandma's house, and her grandma would look at her once and declare, *"Chile, you don got yo'self pregnant!"* Because you know Black grandmas know everything. She could smell you and know you were having sex. She would grab your hands, see your fingers were chubby and your nose was fat, and tell you that she did not need a doctor to know you were pregnant. Depending on how your belly is sitting, she would even be able to determine the gender of your unborn child. I wonder if this is a skill I will develop in time or have I lost it due to my millennial Black privilege. Only time will tell.

One thing I have learned from having a Black mama is that they will always accept you after they have told you about yourself. Your mother may shake her head in disappointment, call you a name or two, and then tell you, *"Come here, baby,"* and do everything in her power to be the best grandma in the world. Thankfully I did not have a name-calling mama. She has never made me feel like my decisions were subpar, even when she did not fully understand what it was that I was doing with my life. When I told my mother I was taking a break from college, she just said, *"Okay,"* with a little confusion. When I told her I was pregnant, she became quiet. She took a deep breath, and, as I vaguely remember, she let out a little bit of a laugh and said something along the lines of *"I'm going to have another grandbaby!"* My shoulders eased and I instantly became peaceful. As long as my mama accepted me, I knew I could make it through anything. Here's a bit of upfront advice that can save you a lot of arguments in your family: do not announce your pregnancy on social media before revealing the pregnancy to your mother, father, and probably your grandparents first. What are the best options for a pregnancy reveal? Let's explore a few scenarios.

# Lesson One: Do Not Announce Your Pregnancy on Speakerphone in Front of Your Partner...If Your Parents Don't Really Get Down with Him like That

Depending on where you are in your life, you may not be able to gauge your parents' reaction to finding out their daughter is pregnant. If you are married and actively trying to start a family, you can imagine that their reaction may be positive, and so this lesson may not apply. On the other hand, if this is an "oops" baby and your parents have met your partner only a handful of times, read closely, Sis. Even though you may be excited about this news, breaking it to your parents over Facetime or speakerphone and having FBD (Future Baby Daddy) sit right next to you as your mother cries hysterically about how you have ruined your life will probably not be the most comforting for either of you. Your parents will probably be less offensive if you are pregnant by your husband instead of your boyfriend.

Another lesson I have learned in dating Black men is to never underestimate the love a Black mama will have for her Black son. Sis, while you may have been your boyfriend's mother's favorite girlfriend, those feelings can change once you become your boyfriend's pregnant girlfriend. Black mothers have a tendency to be overly protective of their sons. Even though it takes two to get pregnant (in most cases), his mama may not see it that way. If you do not already have a super close bond with your partner's mother, sit down with your partner and discuss what the possible outcomes may be of her reaction to the news. If he feels she may not be fully accepting right away, allow him to break the news to her first. It is his responsibility after all. Then let time do some healing work and try not to take it too personally.

Before announcing your pregnancy to either of your family members, talk about it first. This reveal is a decision that should be considered between you and your partner first.

# Lesson Two: The Big Social Media Announcement

When it comes to announcing your pregnancy on social media, there can be a lot of social anxiety around making your pregnancy public. For moms who may have experienced infertility issues in the past, like miscarriages, announcing too soon may have proved painful. Announcing too late could mean no announcement at all and just showing up to the digital party with a baby in tow.

So, what is the magic number of months at which it is safe to announce your pregnancy? According to studies, your chances of miscarrying drop significantly after the first trimester. If you have safely made it over the ten to twelve-week hump, you can scream to the social media rooftops that you have a baby on board. In my case, I woke up one day and realized I was six months pregnant. While my close friends and family knew my pregnancy news, I had not announced my baby bump on social media. This was well before *Black Moms Blog*, and my social channels consisted solely of a Facebook page with friends, in state and out of state family members, and coworkers. I was tiny when I was pregnant, only gaining twelve pounds, and it took forever for my belly to finally pop. At six months, I looked down and saw that I no longer looked like a skinny fat person, I actually looked pregnant.

I debated for a while: should I just show up with a newborn on social media in a few months? Like, "Surprise guys! I had a baby and never even told you I was pregnant!" No, maybe not. Should I get a fancy photo shoot, or a video made to make a big reveal? Ah, no. We were struggling millennials. Spending money on photos at that time was not a priority. I settled on a blurry iPhone photo of my belly in a gray tank top. No face showing and my long, pink manicured gel nails holding my stomach. My breasts looked great in that photo. The caption read something like, "Welcome to the world, baby girl." Tacky with a capital T.

My suggestion is to be a little more intentional with your pregnancy announcement than I was at twenty-three years old. Do not over think it. You can go all out with the fancy photo shoot, create an adorable video, or post your pregnancy test (clean it first). Another important factor in announcing your pregnancy in the age of social media is determining your mental health prior to the big reveal and the responses of your peers. Once again, this is greatly determined by what life stage you are in. If you are someone who is ready to start a family, your self-proclamation will most likely be met with positive comments and congratulations. But, if you are announcing your pregnancy after miscarriages and are active in groups that focus on infertility, you may receive responses that are ripened with jealousy and sadness for their own misfortune. For those that were like me, young and pregnant, you may experience a little more pushback from friends who don't understand why on earth you would consciously choose to move forward with this pregnancy at all. Your pregnancy announcement will not be a one-size-fits-all situation. It is important to prepare for the responses.

# Lesson Three: Jumping Ahead of the Curve: Announcing Your Pregnancy to Your Employer

Depending on what kind of job you have and where you are in your life, announcing your pregnancy to your employer may or may not need to happen before the big social media reveal. Being a Black woman in the workplace comes with its usual set of complications, but pregnancy is one that is universal to all women. Upon being hired, your reproductive health is already a concern. It has been a debated issue whether employers have reason to pay men more than women. If a woman becomes pregnant, will she continue to work? What about maternity leave? How does pregnancy affect a woman's right to stay employed? These answers are of course decided on a case-by-case basis, but the best way to get ahead of the conversation is to speak directly with your human resources department. Find out what your maternity leave options are, and your partner should do the same at their place of work. Some employers will offer paternity leave for dads. It is a great resource and support for mothers to have their partners home to help in those first few weeks.

Make sure to ask your employer about your FMLA options. The FMLA, or Family Medical Leave Act, was passed in 1993 and legally protects a woman or man's job position and offers unpaid leave for a specified amount of time for qualified medical and family reasons. Pregnancy falls smack-dab in the middle of medical and family reasons. There are eligibility requirements around FMLA, such as hours worked and the amount of time you have been employed at a job. A company also has to employ a certain number of workers, and distance from the worksite can also be a determining factor. To determine your FMLA eligibility, speak with your HR department.

# Lesson Four: Deciding How "Revealing" Your Gender Reveal Should Actually Be

The next key item on the pregnancy announcement to-do list is to let everyone know if they are buying hair bows or baseball caps. Gender reveals have become increasingly popular due to social media. Seemingly gone are the days of sending a pink or blue onesie in the mail to loved ones. Now, parents to be are having larger than life celebrations, shooting pink or blue fireworks, and popping balloons to be covered in color-themed party paper. With all the grandiosity around pregnancy announcements, what is right for you and your family?

There is no right or wrong answer here. Your gender reveal is a personal decision. Some families choose to forgo finding out the sex of their baby until birth, while others move forward like we mentioned earlier. Announcing your pregnancy in the age of social media can lead to anxiousness, which no mama needs right now. So sit with yourself, sit with your partner, your children if you already have any, and decide what is best for you.

In the event that you do find yourself turning to the internet for inspiration, let's take a look at all those mom bloggers out there. Which one is right for you?

# Matchmaking with the Perfect Social Mama

Since discovering your pregnancy, you have probably begun to follow and subscribe to every type of mommy blogger on Instagram, YouTube, TikTok, and whatever else you can add. You have downloaded all of the pregnancy apps and hopefully, very intentionally, picked up a copy of this book. I am sure you have already mentally made your list of things you would never do.

"I will never be the type of mom that lets my child watch television all day long."

"I will never buy processed baby foods for my little one."

"I will never let my child cry themselves to sleep."

Let me go ahead and save you a few *I will never*s and tell you right now that, at some point in your momming journey, you will probably do at least one of the things on your imaginary "never" list. I will not stop you from making it, because it is a part of the pregnancy experience, but you have been forewarned. Guess what, Sis? It is completely okay to break a rule. Parenting is not about harsh definites. It is about learning as you go and creating a lifestyle that works best for you and your family—whatever that looks like for *you*.

Even still, you will most definitely find yourself warped into the land of discovering your perfect mom tether online. What does she look like? Is she a helicopter mommy or a relaxed mom? Does she believe in organic living and breastfeeding until her child can ask for the titty, or is she more of a "wine in a canteen at soccer practice" kind of mom? Let me break down a few of the usual suspects.

## Zoe Kravitz's Mom Is Her Superhero

As soon as you click on her social media page, you feel as if you have been swept up into an imaginary world of sepias, beiges, greens, and browns. Every photo has a fade over it and makes you feel a little woozy. You question yourself. Have I encountered a contact high...over the internet? This mom has managed to make grunge look sexy, she appears to only bathe once a week—preferably in the river stream behind her home, which is a recycled school bus, and she eats kale from her garden which she tends to while barefoot. Her child is normally covered in mashed carrots and only wears a cloth diaper 72 percent of the time. Other than that, you are guaranteed to see him running wild, naked, and free, breastfeeding until he is on his way to college. Her hair is in freeform locs, and she makes all of her own clothes. She is one with Mother Earth. This mom may or may not have a White husband.

The thing I love about earth mamas, though, is that they tend to be extremely nonjudgmental. Why? Because they also want to live their lives exactly as they do without being judged for their decisions. They are normally free loving, probably polyamorous, and live a life that a small part of us wishes we could commit to. Damn those social standards, concrete streets, and television sets! These mamas are on the extreme side of the spectrum, and if you have a phone at all to even look them up online, you probably aren't ready to commit to their lifestyle. How do they have phones anyhow? They are fun to follow and a nice escape from reality. We are living through you, Earth Mama.

## The "What the Hell Is So Funny?" Mama

She's laughing. She is hysterically laughing. It does not matter what she is doing. She is cracking up as she does it. She is rubbing her belly and laughing. She is in the middle of her Lamaze class looking indirectly at the camera, head back, rolling in laughter. She is pushing through a med-free contraction, and guess what? She couldn't be laughing harder than if Dave Chappelle himself was her doula. This mama is your Optimistic Octavia and your Positive Patti LaBelle. She makes you feel guilty for ever complaining about puking up your morning milkshake because life is full of happy feelings and good energy. You are bringing a human into this world! What could you possibly have to complain about? This mama normally falls into two categories:

## Your Religious Mama

She is a modern-day religious woman. We like her because she knows that life is still happening around her and she is not constantly trying to convert you to her religion through her words. She believes that by showing you how wonderful life is, you will see that religious mamas are living life too. She has been practicing social distancing since before COVID-19 took over our lives, and she is a master pro at homeschooling and disciplining. Her children are so well behaved and polite, you consider for a moment, finding God yourself and changing your ways. Every so often, she throws a bible verse at you that makes you remember your own upbringing in church. This is what my own mama wanted for my life isn't it? Too bad I was a heathen.

## Your Stay-at-Home, Content Creator Mama

She actually created the movement of the overly happy mother. If you look at her closely, you can see the vein popping in her eye from smiling so hard. Her home should be featured in *Home & Garden*. Her photos always look like her photographer lives in the basement and is there on demand. She is either well put together in jeans and a T-shirt or you can find her with a polka-dot dress just below her knee. We transported this mom straight from 1962. Her children do daily craft activities, like hand painting, while dressed in khakis and white T-shirts in their sterile playrooms with white sofas. This mama probably married her college sweetheart and is perfectly content with staying home and providing a secure home base for her family.

Do not let this mama fool you though. She is getting to the bag by being the poster child for Black happy families as a top sought-out social media influencer. She can teach you to do the same by subscribing to her email list and paying $999 for her new and improved web course.

## The Feminist Workhorse Mama

A baby could never stop this mom from succeeding. She believes in equal rights, working up until labor, and looking fly while simultaneously being the most badass "mompreneur" or running the next Fortune 500 company. This mama is a literal walking inspiration. We cheer her on from the sidelines yelling, "YYYASSSSSSS SSSSSIIIIISSSSS" every time she conquers a new goal—the whole time doing it with a baby on her hip. Her mantra is equal partnership, but her husband is a complete mystery to us. Some say he funded her startup and she flipped it into a multi-million-dollar business. Others say he is a stay-at-home dad. We will never know. She posts a photo of him once every fifty-two images she uploads to the Gram. The whole time we are left wondering, how does Sis push that Nuna stroller in a business suit and five-inch heels? Goals.

## The "Party like a Rock Star" Mama

We are all subconsciously a bit jealous of this mama but want to live her life at the same time. Sis has found herself after leaving a bad relationship. Self-care is one of her top priorities and she is always bathing and applying face masks. She goes on dates with men in the city, vacations to Turks & Caicos at least once a season, and knows the Who's Who in every industry. Her kid is a walking H&M ad, and they reside in a high rise in some major city. One day she is dating a football player. Next week she is dating a rapper. We live vicariously through her stories of dating as a single mom and how having a child doesn't stop her life. She has mastered the balance between freedom and still being a kick-ass mom. We need tips, Sis. Show us the way.

But then suddenly, she disappears, because what are responsibilities, after all? She pops back up on our timelines six months later, married, pregnant, and on her way to converting into the *stay-at-home, content creator* mama.

· · ·

At some point in your mom journey, you may find yourself morphing into some version of each of these moms and settle safely in the gray area. Motherhood can never be defined but will constantly evolve as you grow. It will change you. It will make you question your choices. It will test your relationships. Overall, do not get caught up in trying to live someone else's version of your life. Just be you. You are perfectly imperfect as you are.

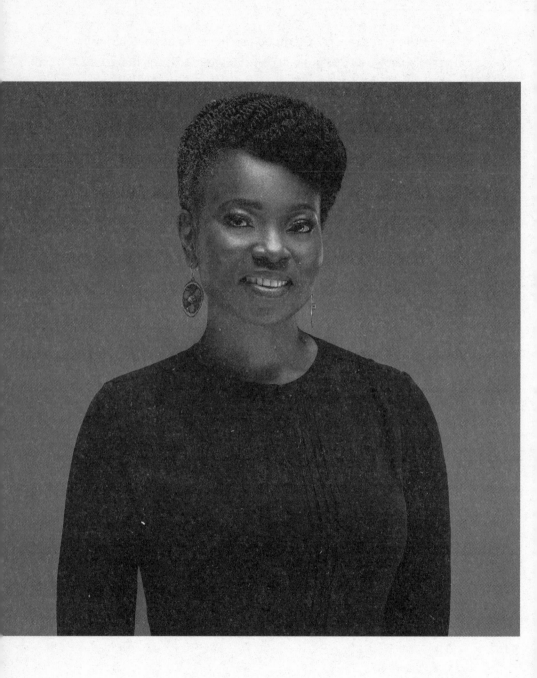

## Chapter Six

# A Conversation on Nutrition with Agatha Achindu

*I have standards I don't plan on lowering for anybody...including myself.*

—Zendaya

**Nutrition is an important part** of pregnancy. According to Healthline.com, good nutrition during pregnancy directly correlates with strong brain development in our children and a good and healthy birth weight. How you eat not only affects your growing baby, it can also reduce the risk of birth defects and illnesses, and can diminish morning sickness, fatigue, and anemia in pregnant women. For moms that are inclined to crash diet after learning of their pregnancy, I advise you not to do this. Speak with your health provider before making any major changes in your current diet. Pregnant women need around three hundred extra calories daily during pregnancy to remain healthy. A balanced diet will always outweigh crash dieting and extreme changes in your normal food routine. A combination of whole grains, fruits, vegetables, and proteins is ideal.

For this chapter, it was important to speak with a certified nutritionist to get her take on how mothers can ensure a healthy pregnancy through their daily food intake.

Agatha Achindu is a wellness entrepreneur, speaker, and educator who specializes in helping American families thrive by transforming the way they live and feed their children. As the founder of Yummy Spoonfuls, a line of fresh-frozen organic food for kids, she's on an unrelenting mission to make healthy food convenient and accessible for busy parents and families. A certified integrative nutrition coach and yoga instructor, she extends her mission further by offering a brand perspective that amplifies her message of whole living for modern times.

For Agatha, eating healthy and nutritious food has never been a trend but instead a way of life. Growing up on her parent's organic farm in Cameroon in West Africa, the kitchen was the hub of activity for their family. Meals were made from scratch with fresh ingredients grown from the earth, and this approach would become the foundation of her life's work as a wife, mom, food activist, and businesswoman. A former IT executive at a Fortune 500 company, Agatha left corporate America and launched Yummy Spoonfuls in 2006. Her goal was to give parents a way to feed their children healthy foods in a convenient way that matched their busy lifestyles. For her efforts and expertise, she has become a voice of authority in her field. Agatha is a regular contributor to the *Washington Post*, and has appeared in notable media outlets such as the *Today Show*, CNN, CBS, *Forbes*, *Fortune*, and *People Magazine*.

As a highly sought after and international speaker, Agatha is known for delivering passionate talks on a variety of topics, including organic food and farming, children's health and nutrition, business development, marketing, supply chains, and more. She has served as a guest lecturer at colleges and universities both stateside and abroad and has spoken at high-profile events such as SXSW, the W.E.L.L. Summit, BlogHer, the AmericaPack Summit, BroccoliCon, and the HOPE Global Forum. She is also a dedicated champion for women in business and seeks to empower them with practical strategies to pursue their dreams without sacrificing their well-being. Agatha's platform represents what it means to live a whole, full, and vibrant life that nourishes the mind, body, and soul. Her burgeoning wellness empire offers something for everyone—from the curious toddler to the wisest elder—and she won't rest until they all have what they need to live and be well.

# A Conversation with Nutritionist Agatha Achindu

**Can you tell me about your work with nutrition and why it has become a pivotal part of your business?**

**Agatha Achindu:** I have spent the last twenty-five years of my life helping families thrive by transforming their relationship with food and self. Nutrition plays such a critical role in the prevention, treatment, and in some instances cure of a majority of modern disease and sickness.

When I moved to the United States in the early '90s, I was shocked to see so much sickness in my community. America didn't look like the glossy images I grew up poring over in the few Black magazines that I could lay my hands on in the mid '80s like *Jet* and *Ebony*. We used to devour each and every page dreaming about the day we would come to America and be a part of this wonderful world.

What I was seeing, in real time, didn't make any sense to me. Yes, there were the beautiful cars, large homes and buildings, and well-manicured lawns on the side of beautiful streets that were mostly free of dust, but something was missing. Where were all the happy people filled with energy, walking the streets and riding their bikes?

My first week in America was such an eye-opener, almost every child I saw had something going on, runny nose, ear infection, skin rash, or a dental issue. It was the same with adults. There were weight, diabetes, and cholesterol issues, and so many people were on maintenance drugs. This was so new to me. We did not have "everyday" sick kids back at home. In most communities, there was that one child born with a defect that everyone knew, but the rest of the kids, most often poor, were healthy and happy.

Then I went to my first American grocery store and it all made sense. There was not any food. Tucked in a little corner of a large supermarket were a few shelves with fresh produce, while the rest of the store was filled with rows of packaged goods, from boxed cereals to all types of canned and frozen foods, some with two to three years of shelf life. Prior to arriving in America, the only packaged foods I knew were peanut oil, butter, tomato paste, and sardines. Everything else we ate came from either our farm or the local market. For someone who had never eaten canned food in her whole twenty-three years on Mother Earth, opening a can of corn and being hit with the most offensive smell did it for me.

As an outsider looking in, it was easy for me to see why there was so much sickness in my community. I was not surprised when I found on the CDC website that seven out of the top ten causes of death are nutrition and lifestyle related.

I started helping friends make little changes to their everyday lives, with an emphasis on food. I knew there was an immediacy that they could easily experience, and it worked. I became the go-to person when someone wasn't feeling their best. I would get calls from people I have never met. I remember one phone call: "My child has an ear infection and we have been to the pediatrician twice already. A friend said I should give you a call." Calls like these became my new normal, I started hosting free workshops, talking to parents about the importance of nutrition, and teaching them small changes they could make for big results.

We live in a society that doesn't invest in preventative care; so much money is in sickness care. I have made it my life's work to make healthy living accessible to all, and most importantly to create awareness around the fact that we are not helpless victims of sickness and diseases; we have control over it in our daily choices. Helping families restore full health and total happiness through my "Life Unprocessed" coaching classes is a continuation of my life's work. I risked everything we owned to launch the very first nationally distributed organic food for kids, food made like parents would at home if they had the time and knowledge, without any preservatives or additives— because I know healthy food must be convenient.

Nutrition is a huge part of total wellness; it is a crucial part of my brand. Every day, I teach others how to eat, love, and be happy—because good health should be accessible to everyone.

**Why is nutrition so important for pregnant women?**

**AA:** I want to start with this quote from Dr Maya Angelou: "I did then what I knew how to do. Now that I know better, I do better."

I believe with all my heart that we as mothers want what is best for our children. As a mother and an integrative nutritionist, I cannot stress enough the importance of nutrition from the moment you considering becoming pregnant. Do not wait until you are pregnant. This is so important to ensure adequate nutrition for the developing fetus from day one. The first few weeks after conception are a critical period of growth. If you were not already eating well, you are unintentionally starting your child off with a slight disadvantage.

Take a deep breath, close your eyes for a moment, and think of the miracle that is happening to you—the gift of new life. Imagine how many women would give everything they have to trade places with you; open your eyes, touch that beautiful belly, and give thanks that, despite it all, you have been chosen to birth new life. *You* have been chosen to love and protect this new being that is growing in your womb, and you will do everything in your power to make it a beautiful, loving, and nurturing home.

Building healthy cells starts in a mother's womb. The embryo needs the best nutrients, free of harmful toxins. Close your eyes again for another minute and imagine your baby developing in that beautiful mama belly, visualize as certain parts of the fetus are being developed—think of your baby's brain being constructed, your baby's nervous system, your baby's circulatory system, and the digestive system all going through gestation one tiny piece at a time. All this amazing growth is happening in real time, and the food you eat has a lot to do with it.

If essential raw materials are not available during this critical time, any of these systems you are visualizing can be affected, perhaps manifesting as heart defects, digestive problems, lower IQ, or ADD. While today we all know about genetic defects, we need to start paying attention to defects that result from building a baby in an unhealthy environment, starved of the nutrients it needs to thrive from day one.

I started preparing my body the day we decided we would try for our youngest. I gave up alcohol, no antibiotics, and no prescription medication. I completely eliminated sugary drinks. It was the healthiest I have ever been, from the food I ate to my daily practices. I started taking a folic acid and iron supplement. It took about a year for me to finally get pregnant. Our youngest is fifteen years old today. He has never had an ear infection or suffered from any cavities. He was that child who flew through daycare without catching every viral bug floating around. I am grateful to God that he is such a vibrant and healthy gentleman. I attribute his health today to the effort that went into preparing a healthy womb for him from day one. Do all that you can to prioritize nutrition during pregnancy without worries. Do not beat yourself up. My hope is that you feel empowered with this knowledge. We are mothers. We have no time for guilt. We learn and try our best moving forward.

**Are there any risks that Black women face more than other races when it comes to our health and pregnancy? How do the foods we eat affect these risks?**

**AA:** Unfortunately, yes, which is why this book is such a useful tool for Black and Brown women. Statistics show that women who are not adequately nourished during pregnancy are more likely to be ill while pregnant and have a higher risk of premature birth and miscarriage. They also have an increased risk of developing conditions that include but are not limited to anemia, infection, tiredness, preeclampsia, and maternal obesity. A study by the University of Pittsburgh School of Health Sciences found that Black, Hispanic, and less-educated women consume a less nutritious diet than their well-educated, White counterparts in the weeks leading up to their first pregnancy. This makes us a high-risk group and is a determining factor in why we need to prioritize nutrition.

The good news is this can be corrected by a change of diet. I know we hear the phrase often, "You are eating for two"; I believe it undermines the importance of the moment. There is more to it than just eating for two. You are eating for your life and that of your growing baby. Your body is going to need more of the right nutrients to ensure you and the baby are healthy and happy instead of constantly sick, tired, and irritated during these nine months. There is an urgency during this period that is completely in your hands. Even if you are on food stamps, you can make it work. I know that having this knowledge will empower and provide the tools you need to choose better for you and your baby. Make choices that breathe life into your beautiful body and support you and your child at a time when you need it the most.

Eating a balanced diet, rich in high-quality, minimally processed foods, including:

- Whole grains
- Fruits (fresh or frozen)
- Vegetables (fresh/frozen)
- Legumes
- Nuts/seeds
- Good-quality meats/ low-mercury fish

Avoid empty caloric, overly processed foods that deplete your body of its nutrients, like:

- Refined sugar
- Refined grains
- Processed fats and oil
- Modern milk

If you are not cooking your meals or buying from a trusted person at your local farmers market or neighborhood joint, make it a habit to read the label, keep an eye on the four ingredients here, and don't eat any food with ingredients you can't pronounce or recognize, when in doubt, check Google.

**How do the foods we eat affect our babies after they are born and breastfeeding?**

**AA:** A study published in *ScienceDaily* suggests a poor diet during pregnancy may have a long-term impact on a child's health. Mothers who eat an unhealthy diet during pregnancy may be putting their children at risk of developing long-term, irreversible health issues including obesity and raised levels of cholesterol and blood sugar, according to research.

A healthy diet in preconception and during pregnancy have been linked to many benefits including reduced risks of preterm birth and fetal growth restriction. A study by researcher Susan E. Ozanne, a clinical biochemist with the University of Cambridge in Great Britain, claims eating a healthy diet during pregnancy—rather than one full of fat and sugar—can increase the baby's lifespan by 50 percent or more.

Today we know that every single cell, organ, and system inside an unborn baby comes mostly from the food the mother eats before and during pregnancy. Nutrition during this "season" is a critical determinant of a baby's health. It is not surprising to see studies attributing childhood diseases to bad eating habits and longevity to good eating habits.

I know we all cannot wait to snap back to our pre-pregnancy glow and drop the baby-making weight. If you are breastfeeding, you want to continue making healthy choices. Remember your diet and breast milk (liquid gold) are closely intertwined. Your daily choices of the food you eat affect your breast milk quality and subsequently your little infant who is nursing.

Short story: I want to share this right now since no one ever told me—not my mother or my aunties. During my first few weeks of breastfeeding, I experienced a sharp pain in my nursing breast. I called my lactationist. "My stomach hurts so much," I said. "I can feel it pulling with every suck! It feels like my baby is trying to pull my stomach out through my breast!" I heard a deep pause. "Agatha," my lactation therapist chimes in, "it is your involution." "My what?" I whispered trying not to wake the baby up. "Involution is when your uterus contracts to shrink back to its normal size after childbirth. That sensation can be quite intense for some," she said. "Now you know, Mama. Go on, tell every pregnant mama you meet; we need to know this thing."

The one year I nursed our youngest, I nourished my body with the best of the best. I consumed whole grains, loads of fresh fruits and vegetables, legumes, grass-fed beef and pastured chicken, organic sprouted tofu, and lots of nuts and seeds. If it could be grown from the ground, I was ready to eat it. I also drank a lot of water. My lactation "magician" told me to drink a large glass of water before and after every feeding. I took that to church and did it religiously. My body was glowing from all that hydration and there was an abundance of "liquid gold."

Remember, as I mentioned earlier, that your food and your child's diet are one. Keep this in mind when you are so tired but have a full day of work and you decide to drink coffee all day. If your baby is acting fussy it might be the caffeine.

I am old school. I grew up on healing herbs, tinctures, and homemade remedies. I am my mother's daughter. If you are like me, please make sure you talk to your health care provider about your herbs. Just because it is natural and you grew up taking it does not necessarily mean it is safe during pregnancy.

**What are a few easy steps a mother can take toward improving her nutrition while pregnant?**

**AA:** Your body needs nutrients to stay healthy. With the precious baby in your beautiful womb, your body needs double the nutrients to nourish both you and your baby, not just in the belly but also their future health. It all starts with what you eat today. The good news is there are some simple steps you can take to very quickly improve your nutrients and thus the health of both you and your baby.

Drink water instead of sugary drinks. Refined sugar is extremely toxic, especially to developing cells.

I am a firm believer in the 80/20 rule. You want to make sure 80 percent of the time you are eating the right foods that support your health. Below are the foods to either limit or completely avoid.

Foods to avoid:

- Highly processed foods: cakes, cookies, chips and fries, donuts etc. (homemade fries with real potato is good)
- Processed meats: deli cold cuts, hot dogs, etc.
- Refined sugar: energy drinks, ice cream, baked goods, cereals, sodas, fruit drinks with added sugar, etc.
- Pizza (homemade pizza is good since you will use real ingredients and whole grain crust)
- High salt foods: read labels, and be mindful of junk foods, etc.
- Alcohol
- Vegetable oils

Foods you need to eat for a balanced diet that will provide an abundance of the nutrients you and baby needs:

- Whole grains: brown rice, quinoa, millet, oats, farro, bulgur, corn, buckwheat, etc.
- Fruits: fresh/frozen (check label when buying frozen)
- Vegetables: fresh/frozen, variety is key; you want to make sure you are feeding the good bacteria that helps with digestion, pregnancy, and constipation. Eat as much raw veggies as humanly possible. The only raw vegetables to avoid would be anything sprouted

- Legumes: Black beans, chickpeas, lentils, peas, soybeans, navy beans, pinto beans, kidney beans, peanut, black eyed peas

- Good-quality protein: Animal (meats, poultry, fish) Plant (tofu, tempeh, lentils, beans, peas, almonds, etc.)

- Good-quality fats/oils: From foods such as avocados, nuts, and seeds, as well as olive oil, avocado oil, coconut oil, ghee, pastured butter, etc. Avoid vegetable oils including canola, which have an oxidative effect in our body and cause a lot of inflammation

During pregnancy, keep your consumption of leafy greens high for that extra boost of calcium and iron that is needed during pregnancy. Sesame seeds are very high in calcium as well. Talk to your health care provider about a good-quality folic acid (folate) supplement.

**Do you have any advice for pregnant women when it comes to their food intake?**

**AA:** Take the time to properly chew your food. I wished I listened to my mother more when I was younger. "Aga," she would call me, "chew your food, your stomach has no teeth." Every time a pregnant mama complains to me about indigestion and bloating feelings, my advice is always the same: chew your food more and let me know if you feel any better.

The simple act of chewing your food properly helps break down larger particles of food into smaller particles, releasing saliva that contains digestive enzymes. This helps to reduce stress on the esophagus and therefore aids the stomach to metabolize your food better. This is one lesson I have been very intentional about teaching my own kids, and I pray to God they are better listeners than I was. Digestion starts in the mouth. The last bit of advice I will leave you with is to please eat more fresh, wholesome greens; half your plate should always be filled with life-giving raw or lightly cooked greens.

*To learn more about Agatha, visit her website at AgathaAchindu.com.*

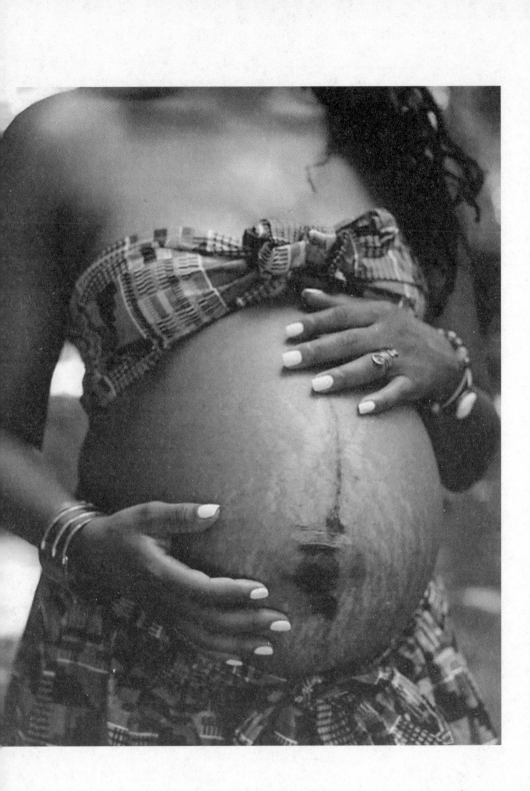

## Chapter Seven

# A Pregnant Hormonal Woman Has Taken Over My Life. I Am Sis. Sis Is Me.

*Embrace what makes you unique, even if it makes others uncomfortable. I didn't have to become perfect because I've learned throughout my journey that perfection is the enemy of greatness.*

—Janelle Monáe

**Pregnancy can turn your entire** world inside out. Babies have a tendency to do that. You may still be trying to hang with your friends to prove to them that pregnancy has not changed anything for you. In your mind, you are practicing your cool and hip mom status even while your baby is in utero. Remember some of those college buddies I mentioned in Chapter One? Yep. Sis was me. I was trying desperately to show them that I could still hang. Want to go to Saturday brunch? Sure, I am down. I will just sip the orange juice instead of the full mimosa, until the acid in the orange juice made me want to vomit. Midday movie? Of course. Until a midday movie turned into nap time before the opening credits even finished. I even attended a sip & paint with a group of friends and missed the majority of the lesson because I had to pee every ten minutes. The worst part about pregnancy pee is that it feels as if you have drunk a gallon of water and joined the Olympics to beat out Usain Bolt to rush to the bathroom, only to see the smallest trickle of liquid escape.

While we are trying so desperately to show that absolutely nothing is changing, our body is sending us on a fast-track emotional and hormonal roller coaster to remind us that actually every single *thing* is changing. Hormonal changes are deeper and more serious than being slightly emotional and crying during a commercial. What is really going on inside of our bodies?

# How Hormones Affect Us during Pregnancy

The truth is, you probably have not felt this hormonal since starting your period in your teens. That is because, as a woman, your hormones are the main component in your reproductive system. When it comes to your reproductive health, you have two main hormones, also known as your "sex hormones." These two hormones are estrogen and testosterone. You can thank estrogen for developing your eggs to maturity in your ovaries. Then these eggs are released during your menstrual cycle. Women also have testosterone which is released in your bloodstream in small doses by your ovaries and adrenal glands. I guess we are part man after all.

There are additional hormones that aid in the menstrual cycle, such as the follicle-stimulating hormone (this matures the egg in your ovary), the luteinizing hormone. Stimulation of this hormone releases your egg (hello, period!). Another hormone, progesterone, works with estrogen to help maintain the uterus lining. Each of these hormones plays a critical role in your ability to reproduce. If a woman is struggling with fertility issues, it could mean that something is wrong with her hormones. With technology and a better understanding of hormones, women who suffer from fertility issues may still be able to become pregnant through in vitro fertilization.

There are two main hormones involved in pregnancy: estrogen and progesterone. During pregnancy, we produce more estrogen than we will ever produce in our entire life while not pregnant. Our estrogen levels skyrocket, which can cause morning sickness, or all-day sickness, during your first trimester. Do you notice that your breasts are starting to get bigger in your second trimester? You can thank your estrogen hormones for that. Your milk ducts are developing in preparation for producing breast milk. In addition to morning sickness and bigger breasts, estrogen contributes to that beautiful "pregnancy glow" that you are sure to get major compliments on. Pregnancy can also tend to clear up acne in some women and cause acne in others. Thanks hormones!

## What the Smell Is Up?

You have probably noticed during your pregnancy that smells that you used to enjoy, like sniffing your partner's armpits, are now not as erotic and enjoyable. Before pregnancy, his cologne used to turn you on. Even the smell of his deodorant reminded you of something sexual. Now that you are actually knocked up, those smells are taking a different turn. Once again, go ahead and send a thank you card to estrogen. Your pregnancy hormones are sure to turn you into a hound dog that can rapidly smell the underlying funk in any situation. During my own pregnancy, I purchased every scent of deodorant for my daughter's father because the smell of his armpits sent me gagging every single time he was near me. There may be many biological reasons why the sense of smell is heightened during pregnancy, but among the main culprits are those wonderful pregnancy hormones. All that additional estrogen is making you a lot more sensitive to smell. In fact, for a lot of women, their change in smell is one of their first indications of pregnancy.

If you are wondering if you can just vote men off the island for the remainder of your pregnancy, let's try a few more things first. When the funky is making your belly flip during pregnancy, try to look for scents that are less harsh to wear. It may be time to put away your favorite perfume and swap out your products for something a bit more natural. Use lotions and body oils that are also not heavily chemical-based. Chamomile, cinnamon, and lavender are good scents to stick to. In addition to using it as a scent, drinking chamomile tea can soothe the belly and relieve gas, bloating, and constipation. Visit your favorite oil lady in the Afrocentric part of town. We all got one in our city, Sis. Support a Black-owned business and pick up something the juju man says will be peaceful for the baby. Aromatherapy is also a good route to try. Get an oil diffuser for your home or office.

You can also keep your windows open to allow fresh air to circulate. Remember to clean often to avoid any hidden smells. I know you would like to use pregnancy to avoid cleaning, but most cleaning products are safe for pregnant women to use as directed, even bleach. Just make sure you use gloves. Even though most cleaners are safe to use, the smell of certain products can make you more nauseous than others, so it may be good to switch to a more naturally scented cleaning solution. If you have a partner, this is also a good time to use the "pregnancy excuse" and hand over the chores to a more responsible party. A woman's got to do what a woman's got to do.

## Tips for Handling Morning Sickness

When I first became pregnant, I assumed that morning sickness meant that my food aversions, sensitivity to smells, and inability to contain anything I had eaten would only be reserved to the morning time. The truth is, my "morning" sickness was actually an all-day sickness. "Morning" sickness is most likely called as such because this is when most women first experience it. You should be aware of what time of day you tend to become sick and adjust your eating habits during this time. Instead of eating a full omelet with cheese grits for breakfast, you may want to eat a more settling meal like avocado toast and fruit. If lunchtime is a sensitive time to eat, try a healthy smoothie. Also give yourself time to allow your food to process. Rushing between meals can cause a bad onset of morning sickness. If you have already been experiencing morning sickness, you know how unpleasant it can be. While most women have morning sickness, for some it only strikes in the first trimester, while for others it can be experienced during their entire pregnancy.

If you are experiencing an extreme case of morning sickness, you may have hyperemesis gravidarum which affects about one in fifty women. You should see your doctor.

FYI from Medicine Net:

> Hyperemesis gravidarum: Extreme, excessive, and persistent vomiting in early pregnancy that may lead to dehydration and malnutrition. It is usually associated with weight loss of more than 5 percent of the woman's pre-pregnancy weight. Hyperemesis gravidarum affects about one in every three hundred pregnant women and is most common in young women, in first pregnancies, and in women carrying multiple fetuses. Hyperemesis gravidarum usually stops on its own by the twentieth week of pregnancy. Treatment of mild hyperemesis gravidarum usually involves dietary measures, rest, and use of antacids. Very severe hyperemesis gravidarum may call for the use of intravenous fluids and nutrition.[3]

Even though you may experience some interesting food cravings, it may not be best to give in to all of them. Food cravings can be affected by low levels of estrogen, high levels of progesterone, and hormonal fluctuations. Think of it like this: your estrogen can decrease hunger, but progesterone blocks estrogen's effect on

3    www.medicinenet.com/script/main/art.asp?articlekey=8058

the hypothalamus, otherwise known as the brain's food epicenter. Instead, progesterone stimulates your hunger. It's your own body setting you up for betrayal.

Greasy foods are more prone to cause a mishap, as well as foods that contain a lot of sugar. Instead, try eating fresh fruits and veggies. Salty snacks like nuts and crackers can also help to settle your stomach and are good for your growing baby. Leafy greens are healthy to eat. The darker the green vegetable, the better. Leafy greens that are extremely good picks for pregnant women to consume are kale and spinach. They both contain fiber, vitamins C, K, and A, calcium, iron, and potassium. Throw a little broccoli into the mix to add a rich dose of antioxidants.

For fruits, I like to suggest eating anything that looks like it's pregnant. Apricots, oranges, mangos, and pears are a great place to start. You can also consume avocados, bananas, and grapes. Bananas may not look like they're pregnant but more like that thing that got you pregnant. Pregnancy humor. You have to love it.

# Pregnancy Skin: Glow or No?

I am sure you have heard it before: once you become pregnant, your skin is supposed to glow like the sun. You can throw away all of your highlighter because your growing baby bump and additional hormones are supposed to make your face dewy, supple, and as soft as your newborn baby's butt cheeks. For some women, their experience may be the exact opposite. Due to the additional hormones, the hormone androgen to be specific, your skin during pregnancy may be more prone to acne than before.

Androgen normally strikes during the first and second trimester, causing your pores on your face to expand while also creating more oil called sebum. Sebum clogs your ever-growing pores increasing the likelihood of breakouts. Say hello to new pimples. To help combat acne during pregnancy, remember to watch your food intake and drink lots of water. Clear skin starts within. You can also invest in a great facial wash like Cetaphil or Aveeno, which are both light foamy cleansers that work well on sensitive and oily skin.

# Hair Growth and Hair Loss during Pregnancy and Postpartum

In the same way you may notice changes in your skin, you will most likely see an increase of hair growth during your pregnancy as well. The hormone estrogen causes your hair and your nails to become stronger. The additional hormones can make your hair thicker, shinier, and cause your hair that would normally shed to be retained during pregnancy. Your hair goes through three growth stages: the active growth stage, or anagen, the transitional stage, or catagen, and the resting phase, or telogen. During telogen is when our hair normally sheds, but because of your extra hormones, this stage is extended to keep the hair strong and healthy.

So, what happens when all those yummy hormones dissipate during postpartum? Your hair sheds...and it sheds a lot. Most women can lose balls of hair, which can start around three months and last until twelve months postpartum. This can be alarming if you are not prepared. So, Sis, I am trying to prepare you. Hair growth and hair loss are completely normal during pregnancy and after birth. Even though your hair may appear to be thinner in certain areas, after around one year postpartum your hair growth will return to normal.

# What Else Are My Hormones Affecting during My Pregnancy?

You may notice a few additional changes in your body during pregnancy. One of these differences can be the development of carpal tunnel syndrome. Carpal tunnel occurs when the nerves are pinched in between the bones and ligaments in the wrist, causing numbness and tingling in the arm and hand. Because of your changing hormones, there can be a buildup of fluid resulting in carpal tunnel. If you develop carpal tunnel during pregnancy, it will normally go away on its own.

Does sitting down and getting up too fast make you feel as if you could faint? This is because of human chorionic gonadotropin, a pregnancy hormone which is also responsible for the nausea you may experience in the first and second trimesters. Your hormones contribute to causing your blood vessels to dilate, resulting in lightheadedness. If you are pregnant during the summer, take it easy. The dilation of your blood vessels can also cause shortness of breath, especially in the hotter months. Other causes of dizziness can be related to your blood sugar, so make sure you speak to your doctor if you notice you are becoming dizzy to the point of not being able to engage in daily activities.

It is important to mention how pregnancy can lead to anemia even though it is not directly related to hormones. Anemia happens when your body is iron deficient because it is not producing enough red blood cells. In turn, this causes a lack of oxygen flow to your vital organs. When you are pregnant, you will produce more blood than at any other time in your life. If you are iron and nutrient deficient, your body will not be able to keep up with the production of blood needed to support your growing baby, which can result in your being diagnosed with mild anemia during pregnancy. Refer back to Chapter One to read about the importance of taking prenatal vitamins while you are pregnant.

# It's Just Emotions Taking Me Over

Eventually, your morning sickness and sensitivity to smells will subside, but your emotions can take a bit longer. Go ahead and cue "Emotions" by Destiny's Child and cry about it.

Ooo baby
And where are you now, now that I need you?
Tears on my pillow wherever you go
Cry me a river that leads to your ocean
You never see me fall apart...

Sis, I know your partner is asking you five hundred questions an hour. Don't cuss him out. As soon as you cuss him out, you will probably cry about it and then ask that he cuddle you. Next, you are going to want ice cream. To be honest, just get used to the idea that you do not have any idea of what you want, except for maybe your own mom. Pregnancy hormones are sure to open up your well for tears and mood swings, some of which you will not be able to offer up a clear explanation for. While it should be expected that there will be some emotional changes during pregnancy, none should drive you to the point of extreme stress and anxiety. If you feel that your mood swings are leading to a state of severe sadness, you should see your doctor immediately. Intense mood swings during pregnancy can lead to postpartum depression. We will talk about this later in the book.

In order to increase your likelihood of a healthy pregnancy, you want to keep a keen eye on your emotions. Your baby feels everything that you experience and is aware of a stressful environment. For Black women, this is extremely important. Data shows that Black women experience an increased level of stress compared to White women. We have witnessed what this stress looks like, sometimes in our own households. If you are a single mom already and this is another pregnancy, worry and stress about bills and juggling it all can lead you into a spiral. Not to mention, the world can already view you as a statistic. Your response to being a Black and pregnant woman may not always be met with positivity and acceptance. In general, pregnancy can make you extremely emotional, but instead of channeling that emotion into negativity, you can practice meditation, proper planning—which you are already doing just by reading this book— and calmness to help soothe your worry.

Instead of being plagued by worry, let's discuss how you plan to deliver your baby. Preparation is key when it comes to childbirth. The more you take the time to plan all of your options, the smoother your transition will be.

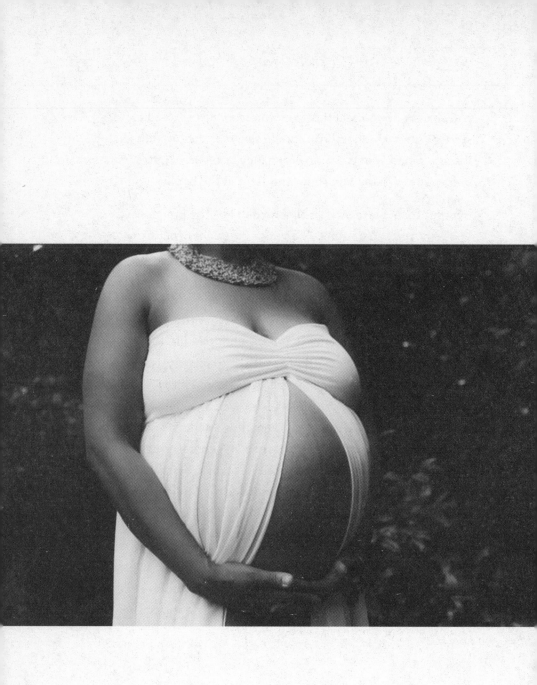

## Chapter Eight

# What Are My Options for Labor & Delivery?

*It is so liberating to really know what I want, what truly makes me happy, what I will not tolerate. I have learned that it is no one else's job to take care of me but me.*

—Beyoncé

**Somewhere in the third or** fourth month of my pregnancy, I concluded that I would have a natural birth. I had little to no reference for the birth process, it was just something that I wanted to do. I was also deathly afraid of needles, and every time I looked up a photo of an epidural, I figured that pushing a baby out of my vagina could not possibly be as bad as being stabbed in the back of my spine. I considered that I would only be in labor a few days at max, and I could walk away from the experience without worry that something would happen to my baby because of the anesthesia. I was twenty-two, a tad bit ignorant, and had never done any proper research on the effects of anesthesia on mother or child. Most commonly, epidurals have minimal side effects, but even having made this decision blindly, I am still content with the choice I made to proceed with a natural birth.

At exactly thirty-two weeks pregnant, I decided that I did not just want a regular natural birth, I wanted a water birth. At the time, my mom tether was definitely an earth mama, and even though I could not birth in a flowing river stream, I wanted to get as close as I could to the experience. My Medicaid allowed for a plastic tub on the hospital floor. Even though there were more than a handful of hospitals in my area, there were only two that allowed water births at the time. My current hospital was not one of them. I made the decision to change hospitals with only two months of pregnancy left to go. I found out that water birthing involved more than my decision: I had to pay a fee, register for a class, and be an optimal patient to do so. To increase my chances of having a med-free birth, I picked up a book on hypnobirthing to learn how I could *ohhmmmm* my way through labor like the White woman on the front cover. I wanted to om. I needed to om. And so, I started practicing my om.

Making my decision to have a natural water birth came without many options. I did not have social media to influence my choice. Birth photography and videography had not become a viral statement yet. I just knew what I wanted and I went for that. When I look back at my decision, the one thing that I am the most grateful for is that I did not pressure myself. I told myself that if I could move forward with an unmedicated birth, then I would do so. If the pain became too great or my baby faced complications, then I would take a different route. I released my own anxiety and trusted my body through the process. At the end of my delivery, I managed a natural birth but did not make it into the pool for a water birth. No matter how you choose to birth your baby, the most important factor is creating the outcome of a healthy baby and a healthy mother. How you choose to birth your baby is a personal decision.

# Will It All Go Back to Normal?

Pregnancy is amazing until you fully realize that your adorable baby actually has to come out of *you*. When this thought really resonated in my spirit, I wanted to time travel back to the days when I believed that babies were delivered by storks. Let me wish upon a star and see what happens...nope. I still had to birth my baby. If you are relatively healthy, your OB or midwife will suggest a vaginal birth. A vaginal birth is when the mother pushes the baby through her cervix, which is softened and dilated during labor, and out of her birth canal. After a mother births her baby, she will birth the placenta shortly thereafter. I am telling you this because no one told me, even as I was laying there and felt this intense pressure and, bloop! Out popped my placenta. After birthing a baby, pushing the placenta out is easy work, but it can catch you by surprise if you are not aware of it happening.

If you are worried about your vagina going back to normal after birth, just practice your Kegels. Your vagina is a muscle, and like any muscle, with proper exercising it can be strengthened. Kegels are to help strengthen the pelvic floor of the vagina by contracting and releasing the muscle. You can do them anywhere and without anyone knowing. Just squeeze in like you are trying to hold in pee and release. Squeeze in. Release. You can practice your Kegels intentionally for fifteen to twenty minutes twice a day for the best results. Birth alone will not destroy your vaginal walls. Your body is made for this.

During a vaginal birth, a woman may have a perineal tear or an elective episiotomy. A perineal tear is an involuntary tear of the soft tissue between the vagina and anus. A selective episiotomy is when your OB or midwife surgically cuts the soft tissue to aid with the birth of the baby. This decision is typically not made until it is time to push during labor.

A perineal tear can occur during the pushing process. It is important to listen to your body and push during your contractions. Pushing too fast or too hard can cause a tear. Your positioning is also important. If you are having a natural birth, you have more options on your positioning and can squat or rest on all fours during the pushing process, which can cause less strain on the perineum. Your OB or midwife may apply pressure or gently massage the perineum during labor to help stretch and support the tissue as well.

An elective episiotomy occurs when your OB or midwife finds it necessary to reduce the chance of your perineum tearing. If your baby is coming too fast or needs an immediate delivery, your medical care provider may decide to surgically cut your perineum. This is where I need you to use your voice, Sis. Elective episiotomies are not routine, recommended, or needed for most births. Talk with your provider before birthing to learn their thoughts on when they would decide to do an elective episiotomy.

You may also choose to have a medicated birth. A medicated birth is when you are given anesthesia to help with the pain during labor. We talked about epidurals earlier in the book, but here is a refresher. An epidural provides temporary numbness to the lower regions of your body. It is administered through a catheter, a tiny tube that is placed in the lower part of your back, into the epidural space around your spinal cord. Epidurals are typically harmless, but some women complain of lower back pain well after birth is over. Even though epidurals can stop the pain of labor and delivery, most women can still feel the vaginal pressure of contractions during the delivery process, which will let you know when it is time to push. If you are unable to feel the pressure of your contractions, your medical care provider will guide you through your pushes.

If you are a mother that has a high-risk pregnancy, your OB or midwife may suggest a Cesarean birth. A Cesarean birth is when a baby is delivered through the abdomen, with surgical incisions made all the way through to the uterus. A mother may be considered high risk if she:

- Has existing health conditions included but not limited to obesity, diabetes, a history of a sexually transmitted disease, or if she is HIV positive
- Is carrying multiple babies at once

- Has had a Cesarean birth previously
- Is over the age of forty

Just because you are pregnant with multiples or have had a Cesarean birth for another pregnancy, this does not mean you have to have a Cesarean birth again. VBAC, or vaginal birth after Cesarean, is a strong possibility. Please talk to your medical care provider to discuss your options.

# Hemorrhoids Are Real

You know what I think about hemorrhoids? They are a pain in the ass! Okay seriously, Mama, that was needed. If we are going to have a real conversation about hemorrhoids, I want to loosen you up just a little bit. See what I did there? Twice! I am an author, not a comedian. Just keep that in mind.

Moving on.

Let's start with a basic lesson on what hemorrhoids are. Hemorrhoids occur when the veins of your, ahem...anus, become inflamed and swollen. Later on, we will discuss fire crotch. Right now, let's talk about fire butt. No one likes to discuss hemorrhoids. They are embarrassing. They are painful. They are also a very real part of life and pregnancy. Hemorrhoids happen when there is an unusual amount of strain on the bowel muscles, which can be caused by obesity and pregnancy. Women can experience them typically in the third trimester and after delivery. Hemorrhoids can be external and internal. Internal hemorrhoids normally do not have any symptoms, but external hemorrhoids can be a pain in the ass, literally and figuratively speaking. They can be itchy, uncomfortable, and cause discomfort and bleeding during bowel movements. Pregnant women can experience constipation, increased blood volume, and additional pressure around the anus region due to their blossoming wombs and those lovely hormones working in overdrive. These are all factors that contribute to your likelihood of developing hemorrhoids during pregnancy.

While hemorrhoids may disappear completely on their own after you give birth, they can also be treated with home remedies if your case is not too serious. It is important not to ignore hemorrhoids, so if you think you may have developed them, see your doctor immediately to prevent any further issues or complications.

Home treatments for hemorrhoids include:

- Increasing your fiber intake
- Drinking more water
- Taking Epsom salt baths
- Using witch hazel pads or wipes when using the restroom
- Wearing an ice pack
- Avoiding straining when using the restroom.
- Not holding in bowel movements (use the restroom as soon as you have the urge to go)
- Sleeping on your side to reduce strain
- Strengthening your anus muscles by doing your Kegels

There are also foods to avoid and foods you can eat to reduce your chances of developing hemorrhoids.

Foods to avoid:

- Dairy
- Processed meats

Foods to eat:

- Vegetables like zucchini, green peas, summer squash, and dark leafy veggies
- Oatmeal
- Whole grain bread

Okay, let's move on with the shit show.

# Can I Om My Way into Delivery Too?

The short answer is, I really don't know, Sis. I would love to say that I was successful with my own oming, but I screamed so loud I also believe that I shook the entire hospital. You can om if you want to. Here are a few ways you can choose to proceed through with your pregnancy and delivery.

## Orgasmic Birth

Supposedly, this is really a thing. Since I know there are women out there struggling to have an orgasm with no pregnancy involved, I approach this method like a strange mythological creature, but they say it is possible. Apparently, you can cum your way right into labor. The mind is powerful, and this seems like it involves the same amount of strength as it does to hypnotize your way into a pain free delivery. It involves sexual stimulation to relax the vaginal muscles and help open the cervix. You can have your partner massage your nipples and kiss your erogenous areas (lots of tongue please!). French kissing and even a small amount of clitoral stimulation can also help. Even though birth may not seem like a super sexy act, women that have experienced orgasmic birth say that the pleasurable experience can be attributed to two main factors. The first is the overall mental acceptance that the birth will take place and that it is important to own your pleasure. The second is the baby's position in the birth canal. Your mom tether, earth mama, probably knows all about orgasmic birth.

# Hypnobirthing

Hypnobirthing falls right in line with orgasmic birth. I have heard of its wonders. Hypnobirthing involves using the techniques of self-hypnosis, visualization, deep breathing, and words of affirmation for pain management during labor. Created by Marie F. Mongan, hypnobirthing, otherwise known as the Mongan Method, works to instill confidence and release the fear of birth in women. According to Hypnobirthing International, their program teaches you to fully trust your body and make informed decisions for your birth. I tried hypnobirthing during my own delivery, and while I can account for certain parts of it, I would suggest doing more than just buying a book. Reading the book taught me how to breathe through the pains of labor in the beginning stages, but having an instructor would have pushed me further into the process of grounding through labor. Go to the classes in your area. Have your birth partner practice hypnobirthing with you. I do believe this method can be effective if practiced properly.

# Water Birth

Water birth involves birthing in a tub or pool of warm water. The water is used for pain management to soothe and relax mama. A baby can be successfully delivered into a pool of water without any breathing complications because your baby will still be attached and receiving oxygen from the umbilical cord. A water birth is best done in the care of an OB or midwife. Water births should not be practiced solo without any professional help and can be known to slow down labor if mama becomes too relaxed during the process. Most women wait until the ending stages of labor to start water birth.

# Unassisted Birth

An unassisted birth, or a "free" birth, is the process of birthing without the assistance of a medical care provider. A pregnant mother will determine her own course of labor and check for signs to know when it is time to push. An unassisted birth should not be practiced by an amateur birther.

*I am not a medical provider. Please discuss your birth options with your OB, midwife, or doula.*

# Where Should I Birth?

Your labor and delivery should be experienced in a space where you feel most comfortable. There are three common places women choose to deliver their baby: 1) at home, 2) in a hospital, and 3) in a birthing center. Determining the location of birth also greatly depends on your health insurance. Most health insurance will not cover a home birth or birth at a birthing center. Due to the possibility of complications, most health insurance providers will only cover births in a hospital.

Women who choose to birth at home normally do so because they prefer to be in a space of peace and comfort. This birth is attended by a midwife or doula and whomever else the mother may choose to have in her space during her birthing process. The type of birth is relatively inexpensive because you are birthing at home and are only covering the cost of the supplies that you need for your birth. You are free to light candles, play music, have a videographer and/or photographer, and have your children, if you have any, partake in the experience. Women who are low risk are ideal candidates for home births.

Birthing centers offer close to the same comforts of a home birth but with a bit more supervision. Even though birthing centers cannot offer to perform Cesarean births and cannot use medication like Pitocin to induce labor or use forceps during delivery, most do offer nitrous oxide, or laughing gas, to calm mama during her labor process. Birthing centers are also stocked with items like antibiotics, oxygen tanks, and a Doppler ultrasound system to monitor your baby's heart rate. Birth centers are also normally within a close perimeter of a hospital in case any complications arise. Only women that are considered low risk are accepted into most traditional birthing centers, and most times VBACS can only be performed if no more than one Cesarean has been performed prior to a vaginal birth. If you are interested in birthing at a birth center, you will want to express your desire around the second trimester of birth to start preparation. The average cost for a birthing center is around three to five thousand dollars in most states.

Even though we have many options when it comes to birth, hospital births are still the most common location for labor and delivery. Hospitals are stocked with medical supplies and are able to quickly attend to any complication that may arise, including a Cesarean birth if necessary. If you are a low-risk pregnancy, it is typical to labor in the comfort of your home until your contractions are around four minutes apart consistently and lasting at least a minute each time.

# A Brief Look into Traditional Birth Practices in African Culture

As a Black woman living in America, I found the history of birth practices very intriguing as it related to our original home, Mama Africa. Black American women are becoming more in tune with their own bodies, working with doulas and midwives, and embracing their tribe of sisterhood to help them through pregnancy, childbirth, and raising a child. The concept of the village is loud and strong here in America. You just have to put your ear to the ground to listen closely.

Upon researching traditional birth practices in African culture, I took a look at two particular regions: East Africa and West Africa. I chose East Africa due to their deep-rooted birthing traditions and West Africa because maternal mortality rates there are among the highest in the world. Less than 60 percent of women in West Africa birth their babies under supervised, skilled care. There may be limited resources in terms of electricity and transportation, and poverty overall is a major affecting component in many areas. Compared to a country like Sweden, where one in every 30,000 women die during childbirth, in Nigeria, that number is one in every twenty-two women.

This is not an argument for hospital births as much as it is for proper education, better resources, and an open doorway to the conversation about birth in Africa in general. Traditions are important. In fact, traditions are keeping some women from the hospital, resulting in a higher mortality rate. Is there a way to bridge this gap, for Western medicine and traditional holistic care to work hand in hand? Only time will tell.

Let's look at traditional birthing practices and how we have adopted certain concepts into birth in the Western world. In West African tribal birth, it is customary for women to birth outside and practice grounding by squatting into the earth while being surrounded by sisters and women. The ceremonial grounding process is tied to spiritual and religious purposes: it connects a mother's ability to reproduce with the earth's ability to grow, bonding both the mother of the child and Mother Earth as one. A stool is used to assist with pushing. We see this used often in natural Western births; the use of birthing stools for a gentle transition of baby through the birth canal by putting mother in the position of squatting likened to that of a bowel movement and opening her body for childbirth.

Looking into East African traditional births, we will focus on children being born within the Kinyankore culture specifically. Herbs are used either through oral consumption or inserted vaginally because it is believed that this will cleanse the unborn baby. Mothers do not typically breastfeed or give a baby their "first milk" to avoid sickness. Instead, newborns are given other liquids to consume. Cord cutting is also performed with a reed, and the cord stump is healed with the mother's and family's spit, cow dung powder, dust, and/or herbs, because it is believed that this will encourage healing.

Caring for the placenta is also of great importance. Parts of the placenta can be consumed to help stop postpartum bleeding, while often the placenta is buried. This relates back to the ceremonious grounding that takes place during the birthing process. By planting the placenta in the ground, a woman's fertility is thought to be restored and her womb healed. If another woman present is infertile, she will urinate over the part of the earth where the placenta is buried in hopes of restoring her own fertility.

In America, placenta encapsulation has become increasingly popular. It is thought that by consuming the placenta, increased levels of the hormone oxytocin will be released and help shrink the uterus. As mentioned in the previous paragraph, in East African tribal culture, if a mother is experiencing heavy bleeding after birth, a portion of her placenta is cut and placed in her cheek to help stop the bleeding. In America, the placenta ingestion is a holistic approach that is supposed to work against postpartum depression. Whether this method helps or not, more women are opting to take their placentas home with them from the hospital in order to bury or eat them. Yum.

There are many ties between traditional African births and our births as Black American women. Let's consider the importance of tribe and sisterhood during our own birthing processes. Who are we allowing to surround us as we squat in the earth? Support during your own birth can make a major difference in the entire experience. So, let's figure it out who will be in your birthing circle.

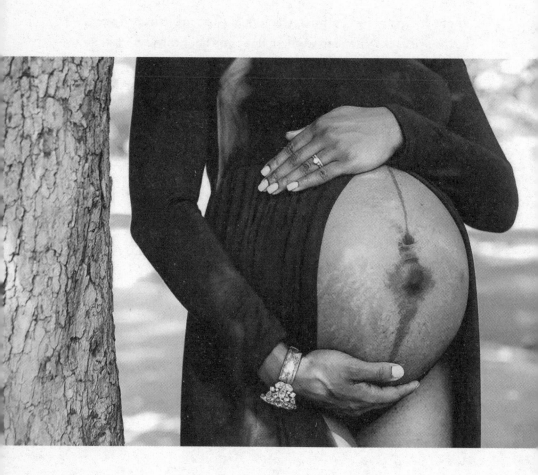

## Chapter Nine

# Why Is the World All Up in My Vagina???

*Nah.*

—**Rosa Parks**

**Moment of truth: I was** not prepared for the amount of people that thought they would be a part of my labor and delivery. As soon as I announced my pregnancy, my best friends, my family members, and even my partner's family assumed they were going to get front row seats to my birth. Outkast's "Elevators" immediately started playing in my head.

"Me and you...yo mama and yo cuzin too..."

No. I was not prepared. At the time, I was barely looking at my vagina. I was not ready for the rest of the world to see what was going on down there. Instead, I decided to have a birth that consisted just of my partner and me. The way I saw it, we made this baby. We should be the one to deliver it. While it was easy for me to tell my friends and other members of my family they could not attend my birth and that I would just call them afterwards, it was a much harder conversation to have with my mother.

She is my *mother*. I realized from the instant I told her I was expecting that she had been planning this moment longer than I could have even imagined. She would call me every day to check on me and offer advice for my impending birth. All of this advice included her being in the room while I was in labor. Each time we had a conversation around this, I was overcome with anxiety. I had envisioned my own birth being calm and relaxing, no drama, no tears, just pushing and birthing my child. That is what I wanted. My mother, while a lover, is the opposite of peace, calm, and no stress. I would be in pain and she would be crying before a tear even left my eye. My mama loves me and because I will always be her baby, she wouldn't realize that I signed up for this and do not need her protection at that moment. Let me suffer in peace.

Telling my mother I did not want her at the hospital during my labor and delivery was one of the hardest conversations I have ever had with her in my life. It was one of those adult-to-parent conversations. Even though I had become an adult as soon as I decided to lay down and get pregnant (*in her eyes*), I made that imaginary line more real when I called her and told her she could not come to the hospital until after the baby was born. She could not be there during my labor either. I knew I would not be strong enough to tell her no once I was in pain, so the best option was to wait until after my daughter arrived. Then I would call her and let her come to the hospital. This was the same rule I gave for everyone. No one arrives until my baby is earthside.

"Hey Mama, so I've been thinking." I spoke hesitantly over the phone. "I don't want anyone at the hospital when I go into labor."

My mom sat there quietly for a moment. "Well, I'm not anyone. I am your mother."

My heart sank. A part of me was hoping she would just say, "Okay, sure! I completely understand!" No, she was defeated. I felt it in her voice as soon as the words left my mouth. I contemplated for a moment. Do I move forward with my decision or do I change my mind? She is my mother, after all. But my mind was made up before I made the call. This was necessary and what I felt was best for me. I was becoming a mother myself and it was important that I start making decisions that best fit my family. This was not about defying my Black mama and telling her no. I felt like I was breaking her heart and ruining a moment she had prepared for her entire life. What mom doesn't want to be in the room when her daughter gives birth?

In the moment of silence that followed after I explained to her why I needed to do this alone, I felt our relationship had reached a new plateau. While a part of her was hurt by my choice, I also believe that she came to respect me as a new mother and not just as her daughter anymore. She knew I had to make this decision for me. It was what I had to do.

Have you decided if your mother will be in your room with you? Your comfort level is of the utmost importance when giving birth. This is the one time to think about yourself. You will be the one in labor. You will be the one birthing your baby.

# Write Out a List

Who do you want in the room as a definite? Who can be spared? If you are birthing in a hospital, there will be a capacity limit on who will be allowed in during labor and delivery, especially if you have to have a Cesarean. Do not think of trying to appease your family and friends—think of your comfort.

The people in your labor and delivery room should be your support system and not your stressors. Let's work on building your ceremony birth circle. Here are a few people you may want to consider:

- Your partner
- Parents
- Your children (if you have any previous)
- Your doula and/or midwife
- A birth photographer/videographer
- A best friend

If you are having a solo birth, then you can scratch the first bullet. If you are like me, then you can scratch the second bullet. If you are one of those moms that believe this is a beautiful moment that should be shared with your child(ren), keep bullet three. Your doula or midwife will be a given. Birth photography and videography are wonderful keepsakes. Do not feel pressured to share online if you don't want to. Just show your kid every time they complain about life being unfair. Lastly, a supportive best friend is always a good idea.

# Your Partner Needs Their Own Support Team

I basically ruined my relationship with my mother for fifteen minutes as I explained why I needed to go through my birth without her. I prepped my daughter's father for this. I made it clear that if my own mother was not allowed in my birthing circle, no one else could crash the party either. In my final hour, all of our preparation went out the window. At nearly midnight and close to eight centimeters dilated, his father walked into the hospital room. I am in that tough part of labor. My contractions are about two minutes apart and forty-five seconds long. I have just enough time in between to barely catch my breath. I completely forgot to pack a robe in my hospital bag (*we will talk about that later*) so I was forced into one of the hospital gowns with only a tie in the back. My entire ass region was exposed. I was experiencing a level of pain that caused me to throw up at any given moment, and in waltzed his father, smiling, happy, and asking me how I feel. Not great, sir. Not great at all. He turns on the light (because I had them dimmed for my own peace and comfort), sits down with his son, and they start listening to jazz music and talking about a helicopter that had just landed on the roof of the hospital. I hobbled to the bathroom, pinching the fabric of my hospital gown together so that I wouldn't expose my entire backside to my daughter's grandfather, and I let out a silent scream.

I learned a very important lesson at that moment: Men need support during labor too. Labor, while it is all about you, is not really *all* about you. You made this baby with someone else. In the final decision-making, it is your choice who you allow in the labor and delivery room. You will be the one going through childbirth. Your comfort is the most important thing. But it may be equally important to discuss with your partner what they may need during that time as well. Make sure you open up the conversation to your partner about what they are looking forward to when it comes to childbirth and what fears they may hold. It will help them to feel included in this process with you. Discuss where it will be best for them to stand. Would you like them in the position to assist catching the baby, in front of you holding your hand and looking in your eyes, or behind you for physical and moral support that you can lean into. Check in with your partner during your pregnancy to ensure that their needs are being met during your pregnancy as well.

As you begin to make these important decisions in preparation for your birth, it is equally important to think about how you will handle your finances. Depending on your insurance plan, your birth can be free or cost upwards of $10,000 (that's an insanely high deductible by the way). Either way, it is better to get your ducks in a row financially rather than try to figure it out later down the road with your back up against the wall...and your baby on your tit. Let's talk about what it actually means to secure the bag before your baby's arrival. Beyoncé has hot sauce in hers. Let's try to figure out how to keep the coins in yours.

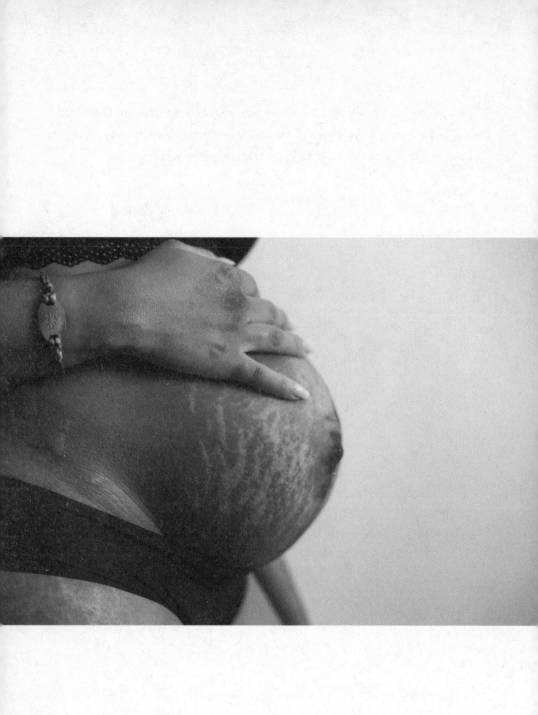

## Chapter Ten

# Focusing on the Bag, Part I: Securing Your Coins before Giving Birth

*You wanna know what scares people? Success. When you don't make moves and when you don't climb up the ladder, everybody loves you because you're not competition.*

—Nicki Minaj

**As a millennial, I am** extremely proud of how financially responsible we have become. If you read broad reports on millennials and spending habits, you will find that we are on course with the generation before us when it comes to retirement savings. Taken from a recent Survey of Consumer Finances, millennial-run households under the age of thirty-five have a median retirement savings of $12,300.[4]

Even still, I am Black.

If you are reading this book, then you are probably Black too. I could spew broad numbers and reports all day, but in most of our families we were the first ones to go to college, buy a house, and marry. We are the first to be business owners, travel the world, and make real change to break generational curses. When it comes to money, we did not start this race with the same economic advantage of some of our White counterparts, but we are creating our own lane in terms of entrepreneurship and financial responsibility.

Here are some numbers for you. According to CNBC, "67 percent of African Americans under the age of forty who earn at least $50,000 annually are invested in stocks either directly or through mutual funds."[5] Even though this is only a 7 percent difference relative to White Americans in the same bracket (their rate was 73 percent), it is the smallest gap in all the age brackets in a study done by Ariel Investments.

---

4   www.nerdwallet.com/article/investing/the-average-retirement-savings-by-age-and-why-you-need-more?utm_campaign=ct_prod&utm_source=forbes&utm_medium=mpsyn.

5   www.cnbc.com/2016/02/05/black-millennials-narrowing-racial-investment-gap-study.html.

I wanted to amp you up a bit before hitting you with a truth you may or may not have prepared yourself for. Babies cost money. Think of your little one as an adorable bill that never stops. This bill begins once you find out you are pregnant and continues on well into adulthood. By focusing on securing your finances during pregnancy, you can arrange for a birth where financial worry can be minimized. You may never completely alleviate the stress of money, but you can for sure prepare for it.

During my own pregnancy, I evaluated my present debt to determine what could be handled immediately and what needed to be set aside for a later date. Like most millennials, I had student loans that peaked over into the five-figure range. While my debt was manageable, I still knew it was important to make arrangements with my financial institutions so that, in the first year at least, I would not be stressed over pending bills.

# How to Find Relief from Student Loan Debt

Whether you have private or government-funded student loans, your options for student loan relief will vary depending on your financial institution. The first step is to make a phone call to learn your options. Some loan institutions offer solutions like deferment, loan forgiveness, income-driven repayment plans, forbearance, or lower interest rates, and may even allow you to pause your student loan payment while on maternity leave.

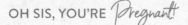

# What Is the Difference between Loan Deferment and Forbearance?

Loan deferments and forbearance are kind of the same and kind of different. A loan deferment can be interest free, so it does not increase your loan amount. Loan deferments are normally a feasible option with government-funded student loans but are left to the discretion of private student loan institutions. A forbearance can pause your student loan payments but will not pause the interest, so your loan amount will continue to grow.

Deferments and forbearance are short-term solutions and should never be relied upon for long-term relief. An option you may want to consider for the long term is an income-based repayment plan. This is when your financial institution takes into consideration your current income to determine your monthly payment amount. While pregnancy may not affect your income right away, if you have never considered trying to lower your monthly student loan payment and have your income considered, this may be a good time to make the phone call. If you have applied for Medicaid or food stamps during your pregnancy, you may also qualify for a loan deferment or forbearance.

# Why Credit Matters

Credit is essential during your parenthood journey. If emergencies arise, you want to be in the financial position to tackle them head on. Being in a good financial position does not necessarily mean having cash on hand but making sure that your credit is in an optimal position for any situation that may occur.

During the time of my pregnancy, I checked my credit report using a free source and found out that my credit was in the low 600s. By the end of my pregnancy, I was able to add an additional forty points to my credit report, putting me close to a 700. Just a few months past my daughter's birth, I had improved my credit enough to fall into the 700-plus credit score range. That was a major accomplishment for me at twenty-three years old. I do recognize, though, that my situation may not be the norm. I paid my student loans regularly, so they were in good standing, and my overall credit card debt only amounted to a little more than fifteen hundred dollars.

I followed a very basic guideline to help boost my credit while pregnant. I had six months left and limited funds, Sis. I was not in the financial position to pay a company to help me with my credit, so I put a little common sense to use and got to work. The first thing I did was review my credit report. I made a note of what was in collection, what had been settled or closed but was still circulating on my report, and what seemed to be inaccurate. Any debt that was inaccurate, I put in dispute. Any debt that had been settled or closed, I put in dispute. Basically, I put everything in dispute. Of the companies where debts had been closed or settled, even though they were legally able to still report to the credit bureau, most agreed to remove the negative items. This resulted in a very quick boost in score. Once this was handled, I took a deep breath and called the collection agencies that were reporting all of my missed payments each month. I set up a payment arrangement with some, and for the smaller accounts, I paid them off right there on the spot. In just a few months, all of my past debts had either been paid off or were now reporting as being paid on time. Who knew accepting responsibility as an adult could feel so rewarding? This felt good.

Before I move on, I just want to mention that I am not a credit professional. These are merely suggestions that you can put into place. I am also here to remind you that getting a grip on your finances will play a crucial role in your parenting style. You got this.

# Should I Buy All the Diapers Now or Later?

I always joke and say that when I turned eighteen years old and moved away to attend college, I faced less financial burden than I did as a high schooler. This was because in high school I had a car, which meant I paid my car insurance and gas. I also had a cell phone, which meant I paid Verizon upwards of seventy dollars a month, and I was responsible for all of my expenses as they related to my toiletries and clothing. Financially, we were okay as a family, but as my mother put it, I had a job, and it was time to learn financial responsibility. Looking back at this time, I am extremely grateful for this lesson. It prepared me for life. Even as a mother now, I look at my daughter with the mindset that I am raising someone who will eventually become an adult. While it is my role to protect and provide, it is also my role to teach her how to protect and provide for herself. We must prepare our children to stand on their own two feet.

After two years of paying my own bills in high school, it came time for me to prepare for my move to Atlanta to attend Georgia State University. The summer that I graduated high school, I decided to keep my job as a receptionist at a car dealership and focus on buying items for my upcoming year of school. Since I was getting rid of my car for my first year of college, I did not want to be stressed wondering how I would get around to pick up items like toothpaste, body wash, and personal hygiene products. Instead, I prepared. I purchased a small purple cubby that I planned to put in my dorm room and stocked it with multiples of my essential items. I bought ten of each product: deodorant, toothpaste, toothbrushes, and soap. I stocked up on my personal items the same way that I stocked up on my school supplies. That purple cubby lasted me well into my second year of college and by time I ran out, I had already learned how to navigate my new city, which wasn't so new anymore. In other words, I had safely prepared for my transition.

When it comes to preparing for the birth of your new bundle of joy, you want to go into your planning process with the same mindset. Do not wait until the last minute to purchase essential items. Essential items are the things you will need no matter what. Because of this, you can start financially preparing to buy them as soon as you find out you are pregnant. In the next chapter, let's talk about the difference between your one-time essential buys and the essential items you will be purchasing time and time again. Have you ever heard of little things called diapers?

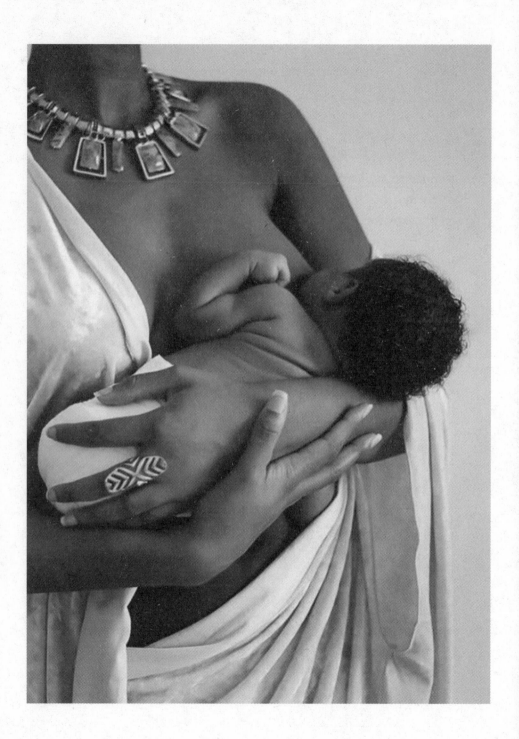

## Chapter Eleven

# The Mighty Powers of the Nesting Mother

*I realized that I don't have to be perfect.
All I have to do is show up and enjoy the
messy, imperfect, and beautiful journey of
my life.*

—Kerry Washington

**There is this very interesting** phenomenon that happens in those last few weeks of pregnancy. You have officially entered the wobble phase of life. Between your belly being a plate for your favorite meals and using your softest pillow to find comfort to sleep on your side, you are most likely trying your hardest to prepare for the arrival of your baby. This stage of pregnancy is called nesting. Nesting is a certain instinctual urge that puts your body in "go" mode for motherhood. It is almost like a bomb goes off inside of your head that finally tells you that very soon you will have a tiny baby in your arms. You may all of sudden feel completely overwhelmed and unprepared, while at the same time running around like a mad woman attempting to babyproof every part of the house and decorate the infant room. During your nesting period, it may feel like there are just not enough hours in the day to get it all done and you will wonder what on earth you have been doing for the last eight months.

Sis. Take a deep breath. Calm down. Every mama goes through a wee bit of anxiety in their final weeks of pregnancy. Are you really ready for this? Yes, you are. To smooth this transition along, I want to introduce you to the baby checklist. It is the ultimate checklist of items that you will need. You do not need to stock up on these items. You will most likely only buy each of these once, which makes selecting which brand or model very important. Hopefully you are reading this book well before your nesting period because the items on this checklist are all essential needs that you can add to your baby shower registry list.

# Your Checklist of Essential Items

## For the House

### Crib

When looking for the perfect crib, there are a few important factors you want to remember. You want to look for a crib that has slats (bars) that are no more than 2⅜ inches apart. The rule of thumb is that if you can put a soda can through it, then it is too big for a baby. Your mattress should not be too soft and should not have any gaps between the crib and the end of the mattress. Read up on the latest safety requirements for cribs. Cribs that have a drop-down side are no longer deemed safe. Most newer model cribs are not made like this, but if someone is offering you a hand-me-down crib, make sure it is up to the proper safety code. Also, if you choose a crib that has roller wheels, double-check to make sure they are properly secured every night before laying the baby down to sleep.

### Bassinet or Co-Sleeper

Co-sleeping is a sensitive topic when it comes to newborns and infants. Co-sleeping is when a parent sleeps in close proximity of their child, which encompasses bed sharing and room sharing. Even though co-sleeping can be convenient, if done improperly, it can prove fatal. The American Academy of Pediatrics recommends room sharing instead of co-sleeping for the first six months to one year.

If you choose to bed share co-sleep, please consider using a sidecar co-sleeper or bassinet. A bassinet is a portable crib for newborn babies up to four months of age. A sidecar co-sleeper can attach directly onto the bed. A bassinet can be pulled beside the bed, but your baby is safely sleeping on their own mattress and within the walls of the bassinet.

## THE DANGERS OF CO-SLEEPING

Co-sleeping increases the risk of SIDS, or Sudden Infant Death Syndrome. SIDS is the sudden, unexplained death of an infant that happens during periods of sleep. Co-sleeping arrangements can contribute to SIDS, but other biological factors such as premature birth, low birth weight, and brain defects can play a role too, and while not biological, parents who smoke can also be a factor. 90 percent of cases of SIDS happen before a baby is six months old. The risk of SIDS greatly decreases after the six-month mark. The American Academy of Pediatrics recommends room sharing as a way to reduce the likelihood of SIDS, but they do not recommend bed sharing.

## Rocking Chair

Rocking chairs are a great way for Mom (and Dad) to spend time with baby in a relaxed position that helps to discourage co-sleeping. Late-night feeding seems easier when you can lie down in the bed to do so, but it is unsafe to breastfeed this way. By using a rocking chair, you have a better probability of staying awake during late-night feedings. Even though Dad is unable to breastfeed, encourage your partner to join you for moral support during nighttime breastfeeding. It can also ensure that mom stays awake during the feeding.

## Changing Table

Changing tables are essential for taking care of dirty diapers on a secure surface. Choose a changing table with bottom shelving to store all of the important items you need to make diaper changing a breeze. Look for a changing table that has secure straps. Even if baby is safely secured, do not ever walk away from the changing table with your baby strapped in. Also make sure to position the changing table near the crib so it makes for an easy transfer. Try to keep changing tables away from heaters or radiators and make sure you have a trashcan or diaper pail nearby.

## Baby Bathtub

It is recommended not to fully bathe your newborn until their umbilical cord falls off. Even though it may seem natural to bathe your baby in the bathtub with you, for safety it is best to bathe your baby in their own bathtub. Babies are slippery! You can use a newborn basin that can fit easily in your sink, or a baby bathtub with back support that fits comfortably within your bathtub.

## Baby Kit (Thermometer, Nail Clippers, Snot Bulb...Fun Times)

At some point, you will need all of these items. Doctors suggest using a digital thermometer for easy reading. Avoid using ear thermometers until after your baby is three months old. Newborns and infants tend to claw at their face, so keep their nails trimmed and use hand mitts for the first few months. You can use a snot bulb, but they are a little old school and are very hard to keep clean. Instead, try investing in a NoseFrida.

## Boppy

A boppy is a baby lounger used for nursing, bottle feeding, napping, propping, tummy time, and sitting up. These are great additions to have to keep your baby close without having to hold them. Make sure when purchasing a boppy to buy one that is made for newborns if you are using it right after birth. Do not allow your baby to nap or sleep in boppy and your infant should never be left in their boppy unattended.

## Baby Swing, Rocker, or Bouncy Chair

I know you think you are going to want to hold your baby twenty-four seven, but a baby swing, rocker, or bouncy chair will be a great addition to your home to rest your arms. Make sure to choose one of these items that are age appropriate, and never leave your baby unattended while using.

# For Outside

## Stroller

The best stroller choice for new parents is a convertible stroller that can be transferred from a newborn stroller, meaning that it is able to hold a car seat, to a reclining infant stroller. If you are pregnant with twins or have multiple children, you can also choose a stroller that is a two-seater or has a toddler standing option. Key features your stroller should include are a locking mechanism to prevent the stroller from rolling, security straps, an over-hood to protect from sunlight, and under storage.

## Car Seat

Before choosing a car seat, read your vehicle's owner manual, which will tell you how your car holds a car seat. Car seats can be secured using a seatbelt or with a LATCH system (Lower Anchors and Tethers for Children) if your car includes one. Newborns are required by law to sit in a rear-facing car seat. You can either purchase a rear-facing-only car seat, which means you will need to purchase another car seat in the future, or you can purchase a convertible car seat which can be rear facing and front facing. It may seem convenient to use a hand-me-down car seat, but for safety reasons, a car seat is an item best purchased brand new. Important features to note when purchasing a car seat are a five-point harness system (which includes two shoulder straps, two waist straps, and a middle strap that goes between the legs), a feature to upgrade or release the straps for more room when necessary (this is important for winter months and bulky sweaters; avoid putting your child in a car seat with bulky jackets), and side-impact protection.

If you need assistance in learning how to install your car seat, visit your local fire department where they can show you how to use one. Hospitals will not allow you to leave without a properly installed car seat, so practice well before delivery.

## Baby Carrier, Sling, or Wrap

A baby carrier or wrap can be worn on the front of the body or on your back. A sling is great for side wear. You want to choose a baby carrier, sling, or wrap that is comfortable, easy to use, and that has a lightweight fabric. If you are using a carrier on the front of your body, your carrier should sit high enough so that you can kiss the top of your baby's head. The fabric should be breathable, and for newborns, having the baby facing inward is the best position. This also comes in handy for breastfeeding.

## BABY WRAPS ARE A CULTURAL EXPERIENCE

Even though baby carrying has become modernized, the art of baby wrapping is a cultural practice that has been done for thousands of years. In African tradition, mothers have used fabric to wrap their babies securely to their bodies. Nigerian women use a rectangular piece of cloth called an "iro," combined with an additional optional piece of fabric called an "oja" for reinforcement. In African culture, babies are carried around the back with their legs placed on either side of their mother. The legs are secured in the fabric so as to not hang or swing too loosely, which can cause a lack of blood circulation to the lower part of the legs and feet.

Baby wearing has many benefits, including but not limited to freeing the mother's hands to do other tasks as well as releasing the hormone oxytocin, which can promote milk production and "let-down" through bonding and skin-to-skin contact.

*Please consult a professional before wearing your baby in a nontraditional baby wrap to ensure your baby is safe and secure.*

# For Mom

## Breast Pump: Manual and Electric

If you are planning to breastfeed, a breast pump, both manual and electric, is an essential item. Breast pumps allow for breast milk to be stored and consumed later by the baby without nipple-to-mouth contact. Breast pumps are a great way to include your partner in feedings to increase bonding and allow mom a time to rest. If you are aching for that glass of wine after pregnancy, you can use stored milk collected through your breast pump to feed your baby.

When choosing a breast pump, you should consider factors like budget, when and if you plan to go back to work, plus the size and bulkiness of your breast pump. While electric breast pumps can be heavier and more expensive, they do tend to get the job done faster and more efficiently. Battery-operated breast pumps are also a good alternative to use in the workspace. They can have the power of an electric breast pump without taking up all the space. Manual breast pumps work with a hand pump and some are even small enough to fit in your diaper bag, which can be great for travel or days out.

If you plan to use a breast pump, you should also purchase milk storage bags.

## Diaper Bag

Becoming a mom means trading in your cute, tiny handbag for a more useful diaper bag. Believe me, Sis, do not try to cut corners on choosing an efficient diaper bag.

There are three popular styles of diaper bags. A messenger diaper bag is worn with the strap across the chest from shoulder to hip and is very modern. A great messenger diaper bag should also be convertible for multi-use wear. These bags are dad friendly, normally very slim, and are easy to access. Messenger diaper bags are considered essential diaper bags because they do not have a lot of room, which means they are useful for one-day travel, containing your basic items like wipes, diapers, and bottles.

A tote diaper bag comes with all of the bells and whistles you would expect with a traditional diaper bag. These diaper bags tend to be a lot bulkier, and for good reason—you can carry your baby's entire room in them. Tote diaper bags are what you send to grandma's house. Tote diaper bags have multiple compartments for a change of clothes, breast pump, a changing pad, multiple bottles, and toys. These bags are heavier and are great to have packed as a standby bag in case you need to grab a diaper bag and jump in the car for a trip.

A backpack diaper bag is a favorite for dads. Backpack diaper bags are more discreet, free up the arms and hands, and evenly distribute weight across the body for less strain on the back. Because they tend to be much slimmer than a traditional diaper bag, there are plenty of compartments for organized space.

Choose a diaper bag that is easy to wipe down for cleaning and which is gender neutral. Chances are you won't be the only one carrying your diaper bag, and Dad may feel more comfortable with a bag that fits his style rather than a hot-pink diaper bag with a floral design.

Now that we have discussed your essential one-time buy checklist, let's focus on your other essential checklist.

These are items that you will need to purchase in bulk or on numerous occasions.

# The Other Checklist for Essential Items

## Diapers! Diapers! And More Diapers!

From the moment you find out you are pregnant, you should go ahead and start a savings account for diapers. On average, a baby from zero to six months goes through around eight to twelve diapers a day. That is around 300 diapers a month! A baby from six to twelve months averages eight diapers per day, or 240 diapers per month. When purchasing diapers, you want to stock up but not overbuy. Your babe will zoom through sizes quickly, so do not overspend on one size of diapers. Instead, try to buy diapers on a month-to-month basis rather than trying to buy enough diapers for the entire year.

There are two main types of diapers: disposable (which also includes eco-friendly disposable diapers) and cloth diapers. If earth mama is your tether, then cloth diapers are right up your alley. Disposable diapers though, are completely safe. They are made from synthetic material and a nontoxic, absorbent, layered compound called sodium polyacrylate. Eco-friendly disposable diapers are very similar but free of dyes, chlorine, latex, fragrance, and lotions. They are normally made from biodegradable and renewable materials. If your baby has sensitive skin, eco-friendly diapers may be the way to go.

Cloth diapers can come flat or pre-folded. Modern cloth diapers don't have the large safety pins older generations used to have and instead come with snaps. These are reusable, machine washable, and adjustable. Cloth diapers can cost more up front but save you a ton in the long run. If you are looking for fun Afrocentric cloth diapers, there are plenty of Black-owned business mamas out there that make them.

## Wet Wipes

Wet wipes are any mama's best friend. You can use them for the face, hands, and bottom. Try to stick to wet wipes that do not contain any fragrance. Your baby already smells like a baby. You do not need fragrance to add to that sweet scent.

## Onesies

Here is a very sound piece of advice: do not overspend on onesies. Onesies will be a magnet for smashed peas, baby throw-up, and a whole lot of slobber. Keep it simple with cotton onesies. These are easily tossable and do not cost a ton of money.

## Burpie Cloths

Burpie cloths are essential to catch the baby spit-up you are trying to save your onesies and your own clothing from. Burpies are used to do exactly that, burp the baby. You sling them over your shoulder and burp your baby after a bottle or breast. If your infant has overeaten, there may be a bit of upchuck that accompanies their burp. Burpie cloths are also important to avoid friction between your clothing and your baby's face. Drape them over your clothing before laying your child on your shoulder or holding them in your arms.

## Bottles and Nipples

If you want to give your actual nipples a rest from breastfeeding, you want to invest in some good nipples...and bottles. You probably won't look at baby bottles the same after this. Of course, they all appear to be equal. Then you wonder: why are there so many different versions of bottles and nipples? Baby bottles can be plastic, glass, stainless steel, or even disposable. Depending on your lifestyle, one bottle can be better for you than another.

For my eco-friendly mamas, you want to invest in glass or stainless-steel bottles. Stainless-steel bottles are very reliable, will not break, and are extremely sturdy. Glass bottles do run the risk of breaking but are great for the environment and do not contain BPA, or bisphenol A. They are also recyclable. If you are worried about breaking your glass bottles, you can purchase a plastic sleeve to use as a cover. Plastic bottles are a normal course of purchase for most moms, but you want to make sure you are buying your plastic bottles brand new. Hand-me-down bottles can contain BPA, an industrial chemical used to make some plastics and resins. BPA is extremely controversial, with some scientists saying it is harmless while others claim it is harmful. BPA can mimic the hormone estrogen and can be broken down and mixed into food and drink components. Disposable bottles are made with a plastic sleeve inside of the bottle for one-time usage. The liner helps prevent air bubbles by collapsing as your baby drinks. Less air bubbles means less gas, which ultimately saves your tiny tot from an upset stomach, burping, and flatulence.

Nipples are equally as important as the bottle because they work to mimic your actual nipple. If you have a breastfed baby, the wrong nipple can completely throw off the bottle-feeding process. Nipples can be either latex or silicone. Latex nipples, while softer and more flexible, can be problematic if your baby has a latex allergy. Silicone nipples have a better shape and are longer lasting but can also be a bit pricier. You can try different shapes of nipples to match the actual shape of your breast. Wide and flat nipples mimic the mother's breast more than dome-shaped nipples. As your baby grows, so will the size of their bottle nipple. Smaller-holed nipples release a slower flow and larger-holed nipples release a faster flow and more milk. If your baby is spitting up and choking while drinking, you may want to reduce the size of your nipple.

## Pacifiers

Pacifiers can be a controversial buy. When used too long, pacifiers can cause teeth to grow in bucked. We all know someone with bucked teeth. It is not an easy life. They also do exactly as they are called, pacify. Babies and parents alike can become dependent on their magical powers, and breaking a baby away from their pacifier can prove to be quite the challenge. Pacifiers are made of silicone or latex and mimic the mother's nipple for soothing. There hasn't been any scientific proof that pacifiers cause nipple confusion, but if you are worried about this problem, wait to introduce pacifiers until after your baby is at least one month old.

## Baby Creams and Lotions

As Black people, we love our creams, shea butters, coconut oils, and body lotions. When it comes to your baby, though, you want to stick to the essentials. Before applying shea butter or coconut oil to your baby's skin, make sure you have an allergy test done at your pediatrician's office. Your baby is already soft. There is not much of a need to make your newborn softer. Take it easy on the creams and choose a light, neutral oil instead. Check with your doctor before using any oil on your baby's skin—this includes diaper rash cream.

Here's a tip, if your baby experiences cradle cap, which is a patchy and scaly crust on the scalp caused by the skin's overproduction of oil, squeeze a little breast milk on it. If the problem has not started to resolve itself in a few days, then consult with your doctor before starting any treatment.

If you have been tallying up how much all of this will cost, I suggest giving yourself a break and adding most of these items to your baby shower registry list. In the next chapter, we will talk about what you should (and should not) expect from your baby shower.

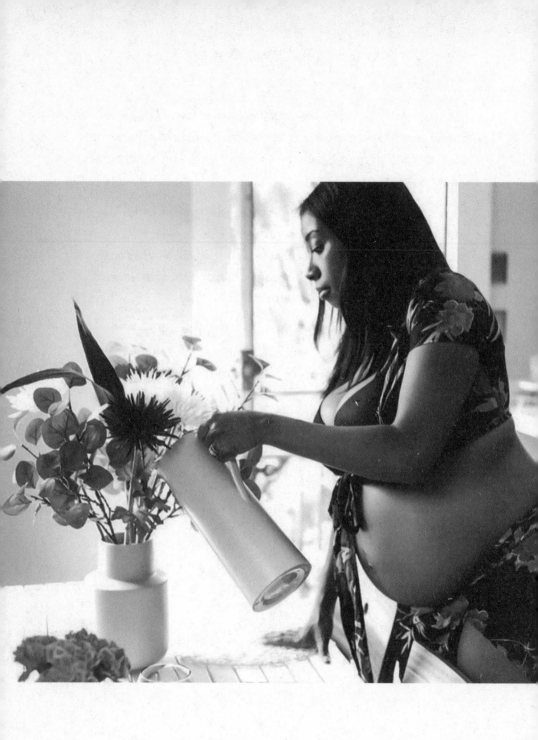

## Chapter Twelve

# Party Party Party... Like a Pregnant Rockstar

*Everything is worth it. The hard work, the times when you're tired, the times where you're a bit sad, in the end, it's all worth it because it really makes me happy. There's nothing better than loving what you do.*

—Aaliyah

**If you have been counting** down the days to when you can finally party again, you are almost there, Sis! You have officially made it to your baby shower. A baby shower is a party that celebrates your introduction into motherhood. Some women use baby showers to scout baby names, collect items for the nursery, and to play fun games with their family and friends.

Celebrations around the births of babies are documented as early as the Egyptian days, but it was not until after World War II that mothers began celebrating the birth of their babes before their actual delivery date. The surge of pregnancy in that time—what we now know as the Baby Boom—coupled with a recovering economy, meant moms needed all the help they could possibly get. With baby showers becoming increasingly popular after World War II, the birth of babies is now celebrated all over the world.

In India, baby showers are referred to as "godh bharai," which means "to fill the lap" signifying the placement of gifts for mom into her lap. In China, baby showers are called "red egg and ginger parties," and are held on the first or second full moon after the baby is born. Guests are given a hard-boiled egg that has been dyed red as a sign of happiness and life renewal and are presented with pickled ginger which is supposed to restore balance to an exhausted mother's yin and yang.

Colonialism, as it plays a major role in most African economies, also has a significant influence over how baby showers are held in African culture. Baby showers in South Africa are referred to as "stork parties," giving in to the belief that babies are given to families by storks. This concept began as European folklore. The theory gained popularity in the nineteenth century because of a story by Hans Christian Anderson that proclaimed that babies were delivered by storks and dropped into a couple's chimney.

Like in American culture, South African baby showers are thrown as a surprise to mom and are more about fun and games than anything ceremonial. The most attention is given to the cake during a stork party. Stork parties are a big deal, with specialized bakeries and event planners helping to plan the showers.

So how should you proceed with your own baby shower? If this is not your first parenting rodeo, you may be feeling apprehensive about having another baby shower. There is absolutely no rule that says if you had a baby shower for a previous birth that you cannot have another! Baby showers can be a huge help to mothers to boost their overall morale as they become parents, even for the second or third time, but also to ease financial burden in preparing for the birth of their child.

# How to Throw a Baby Shower

Traditionally, baby showers are typically hosted by a friend or family member for the expectant mother two or three months prior to their due date. This gives mom ample time to purchase any items that may have not been received at the shower and takes the pressure off of having to be out and about during the last few months of pregnancy. Allowing someone else to throw your baby shower also serves as a gift in itself. As an expectant mom, you have the freedom to just show up and be celebrated. This day is for you and your baby. If you do not have someone to throw your shower for you, you can throw your own. More modern baby showers are being put together by mom herself. You should still have someone host your shower so that you can relax.

Speaking of modernized baby showers, in the past, baby showers were typically an all-girls affair. Nowadays, baby showers are being hosted to celebrate both Mom and Dad, with family and friends being invited in support of both parents. Dad is a part of this special day too, and it is okay to include him in the festivities. Dad can also have a baby shower hosted by his friends, and you can keep the two celebrations separate. Men are becoming more open to the idea of having their own parties to prepare them for parenthood as well. There is no right or wrong way to have your baby shower.

Who to invite to your shower is also your choice. You can keep your guest list small and intimate, only choosing to invite close family members, friends, and work colleagues. In the age of social media, expecting parents also opt to have large, over-the-top baby showers, inviting friends, families, associates, and internet comrades to join in on the special day. Inviting more people does not necessarily mean more gifts, and the more people you invite, the more stress and expense you could be placing on the host. Be considerate of the person hosting your shower when creating your invite list.

In our days of social distancing (or if you are introverted), a virtual baby shower is also a fun spin on the classic idea. Create a group video thread, play games, and have your guests mail your gifts to you instead of hosting an in-person shower.

What about decorations? Your host will most likely check with you on the theme of your baby shower. There are thousands of articles online where you can find ideas on shower themes.

Pinterest is also a good source for choosing a baby shower theme. If you plan to keep your shower gender neutral, you can opt out of the traditional blues and pinks and settle on yellow, purple, or white for your colors. Personally, I had a bumble bee theme and a gender-friendly baby shower.

Make sure you have an open and honest conversation with the host of your baby shower about your needs and wants. It is a special gift to have someone else plan your shower, but your personality should also be taken into account. Use your voice and give your host gentle direction by stating your deal breakers up front so that there isn't any confusion. You will both be thankful for it later. There is nothing worse than an overly hormonal pregnant woman on the day of her baby shower. You should walk into the space and feel at ease...and your host should feel appreciated.

Do you want to have a baby shower without all the fuss? Call up your favorite restaurant and make a reservation. There is no right or wrong way to have your shower. Baby showers can include fun games. A few popular baby shower games include "Don't Say Baby!" with pins. Each time one of your guests accidently says "baby," they lose a pin. The guest with the most pins at the end of the party wins a prize. There is also "Dirty Diaper" and "Guess the Baby Food." In Dirty Diaper, chocolate is smeared in a baby diaper and your guests have to guess the delicacy by having a taste!

# Eating for Two...or Fifty-Two

When planning food for your baby shower, you want to take into consideration the length of your party. If your shower is short and intimate, tapas are a great selection. You can choose fruit and vegetable trays, rectangle sandwiches, and light desserts to satisfy your guests. If you are having a more extravagant baby shower, you may decide on a buffet or hire a caterer for individual food courses. You can always ask family to pitch in and help with cooking to save money. Consider dietary restrictions of your guests by providing vegetarian options if you are a meat eater. A baby shower is to celebrate mom, but you want to make your guests feel comfortable and welcome on your special day. The more welcome they feel, the better the celebration will be for you!

Quirky cakes have become a fun addition to baby showers. You can go the traditional route with a plain cake or have fun with it and have a cake created that is shaped like your beautiful brown belly. Instead of a cake, you can also choose to have cake pops, cupcakes, or other specialty desserts for your party. This allows your guests the freedom to grab a treat as they move around the room.

# It's Your Party but Don't Forget the Gifts

If you are incorporating games into your shower like we mentioned earlier, make sure you have prizes for your guests to take away too. The goal is to create a fun environment for everyone. You can give gift cards, bottles of wine, or body care products. There should also be a gift for your host.

What about your gifts? Is there proper etiquette on when to open your baby shower presents? Depending on the size of your shower, if you have a lot of gifts, it may be best to save gift opening for when you get home. If your shower is more intimate, open your gifts at the end of the shower. People love to see your reaction to the baby items they have purchased! Whether you open your gifts at the shower or at home, proper etiquette is to send a thank you card (or email) to your attendees for their generosity.

# Creating a Registry for Your Needs and Your Wants

In the last chapter, you were presented with a checklist for all of your essential needs as you embark on your journey to motherhood. These items range from big ticket purchases like cribs, car seats, and strollers, to smaller purchases like baby bottles, onesies, and baby wipes. Some moms use their baby shower to help with the financial costs of these items by putting them on a registry list. A baby registry list is when you preselect the items you would like to receive at your baby shower and then send this list to your guests. You can register at different places, online and offline. The best part of registry lists is that you can include how many of each item you would like to have, and your list will alert your guests when an item has already been purchased. This saves time and money and prevents your receiving two car seats and four strollers.

Your baby registry list is also a place to indulge in your wants. If you are not comfortable asking your guests for large ticket purchases, keep it simple. Asking for diapers is always a good idea. You can also ask for things for you, like fuzzy slippers, nipple guards to prevent breast milk leakage, and photo albums to store memories. Your guests can also buy you or your baby presents that are heartfelt, like stuffed animals, baby blankets, and clothing. If you would like a bit more freedom with your gifts, requesting gift cards can also save you the discomfort of receiving items that you don't like. Make a gentle request for your attendees to include gift receipts with their gifts in case you need to exchange an item from your shower.

If you are stumped on what items to include as wants, here is a sample list of items you can include on your registry list.

# Another Checklist for Non-Essential Items

- Diaper pail
- Nursing pads
- Nursing bras
- Bottle warmer and sterilizer
- Baby utensils and baby food blender
- Clothing
- Baby play pin
- Baby shampoos, lotions, and oils
- Towels and washcloths

- Baby toys for room and bath
- Books
- Baby night light
- Humidifier
- Nursery decorations
- Baby proof items
- Baby monitor
- Baby laundry detergent
- Baby memory books

You can also request meal delivery subscriptions and house cleaning services. In those first few months, the last thing you want to be worried about is what is for dinner and if laundry has been done.

Once your baby shower is complete, you will have a more comprehensive idea of what items you still need before the arrival of your little one. You will also be able to include some of these items in your hospital bag. In the next chapter we will go over how to pack the perfect hospital bag for delivery day.

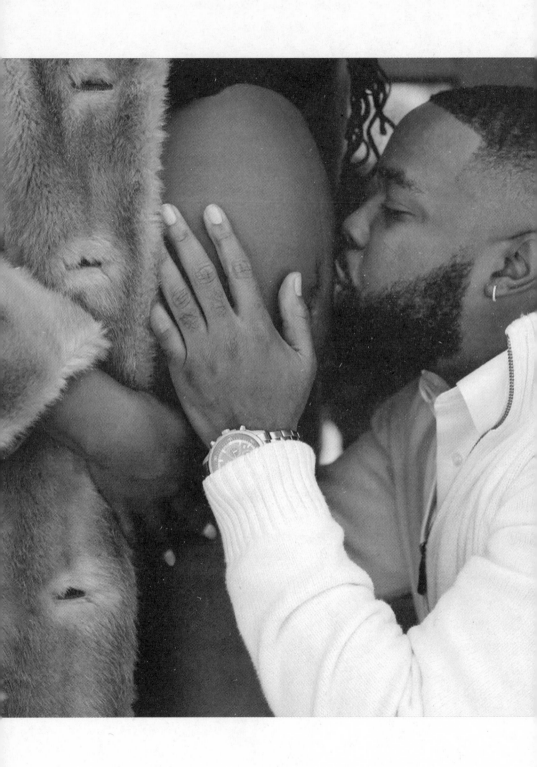

## Chapter Thirteen

# Focusing on the Bag, Part II: Packing the Essentials for D-Day

*I truly believe that if you put your goals in writing, speak them out loud, and work for them, they will happen.*

—**Ciara**

**If you feel like the** previous chapters of your ultimate guide to pregnancy are just checklists, you are partially right. We are finally here—the last few weeks of incubation. In the beginning, it probably felt like this time would never come, but all of a sudden you look down and can no longer see your feet. "D-Day" is near, and depending on what kind of delivery you will be having, you could go into labor at any time. For moms that fall into the high-risk category, your doctor may have scheduled a C-section or induction, or you may have chosen to have an elective C-section, which is a C-section for nonmedical reasons. If you are in good health and are low risk, you are probably sitting here tapping your feet and waiting patiently for labor to start. In the next chapter, we will discuss what signs to look out for to know if you are in labor and when you should head to the hospital.

As you wait out your last few weeks of pregnancy, now would be a great time to make sure to handle any last-minute details or tasks before your baby's arrival.

- Is your nursery fully set up?
- Has your home been deep cleaned?
- Are your bills set for autopay for next month?
- Have you turned in all last-minute work assignments?

Your car seat should be properly installed in your vehicle and you should be comfortable with placing it in and taking it out. Your plan for after leaving the hospital should also be in place. If you have parents or in-laws coming in to help you with your newborn, make sure the room is set up for them, with clean sheets and towels set aside, and that you have a key made so that they can come and go as they please.

**Short story intermission:** Towards the end of my pregnancy, my partner and I moved into a new home to prepare for our baby. We kept putting off the appointment to have the gas turned on and somehow it was scheduled on the day I went into labor. The technician climbed into the attic to turn the breaker and stepped on a soft spot in the ceiling which caused a huge crack down the center of our hallway. I was in active labor, contracting every seven minutes or so, and our ceiling looked like it wanted to cave in. I share this story as a cautionary tale. Handle yo' business.

So, what's next? Let's talk about preparation of your hospital bag. Most women pack their hospital bag around thirty-six weeks. If you are a left-brain thinker, you will probably have the urge to pack two or three hospital bags and place one in each car and your home. Stop overthinking, Sis. You do not need to do all of that. Packing your hospital bag should be simple and stress free. If you are having a vaginal birth, you will most likely only be in the hospital for a day or two after delivery. If you are having a C-section, your expected hospital stay will last on average three to four days after birth. Let's be logical about this and create yet another essential checklist. We are going to break down your essential items into three categories: mom, baby/ies, and your partner.

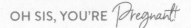
# Essential Items for Your Hospital Bag

## For Mom

### Identification

It may feel easy to lose your head when you go into labor. Hopefully after reading your guidebook, you at least remember to grab your ID, insurance card, and any other mandatory forms the hospital or birthing center has required that you have filled out.

### Birth Plan

This is where your birth plan gains all of its superpowers. Make sure you print out a few copies—one for your doctor and nurses, one for your birth worker if you have one, and one for your partner. For good measure, I would print out another to just tape above your hospital bed.

### Comfortable Clothes to Labor and Leave

Of course, the hospital will provide you a large nightgown with only one tie in the back which conveniently exposes your entire backside. If that works for you then you are all set here. A little secret, this probably won't work for you. Bring your own nightgown and robe. You most likely won't be able to wear shorts during active labor, so grab one of those long comfy grandma nighties from Walmart. Pack in nonslip fuzzy socks or bedroom shoes too. You are going to be going through the Olympics and your body may go through an array of temperature extremes ranging from hot flashes to chills. Pack a separate outfit for leaving the hospital. Choose something breathable and not too tight.

## Toiletries

I cannot stress the importance of bringing your own toiletries. Pack in your shea butter, massage oils, your own soap, head scarves, and lip balm. Do *not* forget the lip balm. Lip balm is one of those special items that you don't realize how important it is until it is gone. Don't find out on your labor day.

## Electronics

Earlier in the book I told you the importance of having a birthing playlist ranging from Beyoncé to 2 Chainz. This playlist will not mean much if your phone, tablet, or computer is not charged. Pack your necessary electronics *and* their chargers. If you are delivering in a birthing center, they may allow you to bring a small Bluetooth speaker or provide their own.

## A Good Book

I know you think you may not have any downtime for reading but you will be surprised. Bring a good book just in case. You can always pack this book too. I'm just saying.

## Maternity Underwear

They are big. They are intimidating. At least they are yours. The hospital will provide you with disposable maternity underwear, but a gentle suggestion is to buy your own. Your lady parts will be sensitive after birth. Be gentle with her. Postpartum underwear can be "period panties"—cotton underwear we don't care much about, disposable briefs, or light compression underwear. The hospital will also provide you with postpartum pads. You can use the ones given to you or pick up your own.

## Pillow and Towels

This is an optional "essential" item. The hospital or birthing center will provide you with pillows and towels, but chances are they won't be as comfortable as your own.

# For Baby

## Coming-Home Outfit

I'm sure you have had your baby's first-day outfit planned for months, but take a few options just in case. Choose two or three outfits that vary in size. If you are birthing in a hospital, you may want to pack an outfit for baby's first photo. Most hospitals have an in-house photographer that will come to your room and offer a photo shoot right there on the spot. Do not forget to pack a hat and baby mittens.

## Diapers, Newborn Bottles (if You Are Not Breastfeeding), & Formula

Your hospital will provide these items for you, but you can pack your own if you have a specific brand you would like to use instead.

# For Your Partner

## Phone Chargers, Camera, Etc.

Chances are, besides being a support system, your partner will be the designated memory collector. Make sure you have your phone charger (grab an extra one for your partner too), your camera and charger, as well as headphones. Your partner will definitely need a quiet moment to themselves at times, so putting on headphones is a good way to peacefully zone out if they need to. Remind them not to be gone too long.

## A Blanket and Pillow

If you are having a hospital birth, there may not be much accommodation for your partner. Most hospital rooms will have a sofa for family or partners to sleep on, but they may want to bring their own blankets and pillows for comfort.

## Food

If your family is already in town, go ahead and have grandma whip up a few to-go containers. While there will be plenty of food for mama to eat at the hospital, most hospitals do not feed visitors or support partners. The hospital will most likely have a cafeteria and your family can leave to get food if you don't pack your own.

## A Change of Clothes and Toiletries

Prepare for the long haul, Dad! Labor can last anywhere from a few hours to a few days. Depending on how far into active labor you are when you arrive at the hospital, you could be sitting for two or five days. Your partner does have the flexibility and freedom to leave and come back to the hospital, but if they don't want to leave your side, at least pack a toothbrush, deodorant, a bar of soap, and fresh underwear.

## Entertainment

This falls in line with your headphones. Bring a book or magazine to take a moment of quiet time to yourself if needed.

. . .

Pregnancy and delivery can sometimes feel isolating for Dad. All of the attention is placed on Mom but what are some things he needs? Our next chapter is just for our fathers. Mama, go ahead and grab Dad and let him read this upcoming chapter with you. Remember that parenthood is a two-person journey and your partner needs support; they're included in this pregnancy too. Our male partners will need a male perspective and support system just as we have our own. Make sure to check in with your partner often and ask how they are feeling during this pregnancy. Believe it or not, Sis, his biggest concern is probably your well-being. Let that man know if you need more support, a foot rub, a bath, or anything else. This is a beautiful time to grow stronger in your relationship and prepare for your family to expand just a little bit more.

## Chapter Fourteen

# A Dedicated View into Pregnancy and Parenting for Our Black Fathers; featuring Anthony Hamilton

*Even to the angels it may sound like a lie*
*For you child*
*He has the troops and extra backup standing by*
*For you child*
*For you he's the best he can be*

—Sade, "Babyfather"

**According to recent statistics, more** than 67 percent of Black children are raised in single-parent households. To our Black men, embarking on this journey into fatherhood probably does not feel as encouraging as you would like. Even with staggering numbers that show the absence of Black fathers in their children's lives, every day we are presented with evidence that more and more Black men are in fact stepping up to the plate and understanding the importance of legacy in family dynamics.

Women, we have it all when it comes to the pregnancy and parenthood journey. We have the blogs and the magazines. The meetups. The books (*you are currently reading one*), the television shows, and the movies. We have our mothers, our grandmothers, our aunties, and our girlfriends. We can sit together and cry vulnerably, ask for breastfeeding advice, and let our guards down to our inner circle and let them know we are truly exhausted. Only in recent years have Black father blogs evolved. Black dad meetups are also still fairly new. As a woman writing this book, I wanted to focus on this phenomenon. I wanted to talk about manly emotions and tell brothers that it is okay to cry, and eventually in this chapter, we will discuss why tapping into those paternal emotions is important. But I want to tell you what happened when I spoke to Black men about what they felt is most important to know about their own journeys into fatherhood. I asked Black men about their emotional needs and I found out that for the majority of the men I spoke with, one of their biggest concerns during pregnancy was their partner. Men wanted to know how to be more supportive of their women. They inquired about what to do when their women weren't feeling well or how they could make them feel better. Men told me to make this chapter less emotional and more factual. I was asked to not approach this section for brothers like a woman. Here is the issue though, I am a woman. My womanness is going to speak to you in some fashion, but before I do let me give the floor to some other brothers to speak to you first.

With the help of a few good Black men, I asked them to spread the word and ask Black fathers this simple question:

**"Black man, what are some of the things you wish you would have known in preparation for fatherhood?"**

In turn, here are some of the responses I received:

*"That I'll never sleep again."*

*"How much my life will change raising a Black boy...looking into society and knowing how men of color are treated scares me."*

*"I was concerned for my partner mostly. My advice is to take care of her. Be there to take care of her needs. Constantly check in on her. Make her life easier, because she's growing and carrying a child. Go to all of the appointments, especially Lamaze. Help her pick out the baby's stuff before it comes. Read parenting books for fathers. Plan on how you are going to raise the kid. Think about what kind of father you want your kid to remember you as. Let her have her silly baby shower and have a good attitude about it. Help her with feedings and diaper changes. Watch the baby at least once a week while she has her 'me time.' Check in with her to see if she's going through postpartum depression. Don't judge her out loud for the silly things she wants to do with or to the kid. Rub her belly with the anti-stretch-marks cream. She'll need constant reassurance when her hormones start acting up and she starts feeling insecure about all kinds of things."*

"I wish I knew how much energy it took. Our son is a ball of energy and wears us both out and still has a full tank."

"I wish I had known how taking care of a child would impact our everyday schedule. You literally have to eat, shit, and shower around the baby's schedule."

"I wish I had known about burnout. You can only be superdad for so long before you have to take the cape off..."

"I wish I had someone to tell me how to respond to the woman's needs as she returned her body to normalcy. How to deal with a woman with postpartum and comfort her. The biggest issue I had was returning to work. Being home for a month was a great help, but when I returned to work I also returned to school. The balance of work and family is so important to understand. Some may think 50/50 is the right split.

"There are no answers. Only questions. Don't beat yourself up for not knowing. No one knows. Just keep trying hard but don't overparent. Leave some things to serendipity."

These anonymous quotes are from the mouths of your fellow brothers. Let's talk about some of the things mentioned.

# Addressing the Elephant in the Room: Raising a Black Body in a World that Doesn't Always Seem to Accept Black Bodies

There is no easy way to address raising a Black child in today's racial climate. With our Black sons and daughters being killed year after year, we have witnessed the murders of seventeen-year-old Trayvon Martin, twelve-year-old Tamir Rice, and twenty-five-year-old Ahmaud Arbery. We are still fighting for justice for Breonna Taylor. For a Black man whose traditional role is to protect and provide for his family, bringing a Black son into this world today can feel as worrisome as raising a son during the Civil Rights movement, during segregation, or during slavery.

The topic of raising a Black son immediately transcends my thinking and takes us to Ta-Nehisi Coates's book *Between the World and Me,* in which Coates writes his very emotional autobiography in the form of a letter to his fifteen-year-old son, explaining to him what it is like to be a Black man in America. He focuses specifically on the murders of Black men in this country: Eric Gardner, Tamir Rice, Michael Brown, and Prince Jones. Coates writes to his son, "Here is what I would like you to know: In America, it is traditional to destroy the Black body—*it is heritage.*" In another quote, he states heroically, "This is your country, this is your world, this is your body, and you must find some way to live within all of it."

I take these two quotes specifically and place them as corresponding examples here in this book. The truth is this, I am a woman. I cannot tell you what it is like to have a Black son and raise him as a man. I can only show you the words of another Black man and help guide you to your own conclusion. Coates's *Between the World and Me* is harrowing. It is insightful, deep, and loving. Painfully loving. It is a book I recommend to any Black man with a Black son. Even though Coates is speaking to his fifteen-year-old son, and you, Black man, are embarking on your fatherhood journey while your seed is in utero, you will eventually find yourself in a position to have this conversation with your child, your Black son, your Black daughter, about what it is like to be Black in America. Make sure you tell them a story of truth but also one of hope, because we are still hopeful. We are thriving. We are beautiful. And even still, we have more opportunity now than we have ever had before.

I am currently writing this book, this particular chapter, during the protests over the murder of George Floyd. During the last few months alone, we have seen even more murders of Black men and women including Sean Reed, Breonna Taylor, and Tony McDade. As of right now, their killers are still walking free. George Floyd's murderers have been arrested, but as we have seen with Trayvon Martin, an arrest does not mean a conviction, so we are all silently holding our breaths waiting for justice to be served in an unjust system. For Black parents as a whole, our worry over parenthood goes beyond the basics. It is deeper than belly charts and food diets. It becomes a conversation about life and death. It is a discussion we are forced to have with our children—to tell them that they do not have the same freedoms to play around, laugh, be loud, make mistakes, have a lapse in judgment, and be disrespectful. That they cannot run free without someone accusing them of stealing something, that they cannot fight back, in some cases that they cannot fight at all. We have to tell them that even on their bad days, they cannot catch an attitude. We have to tell our sons that at some point in their life they will no longer be adorable but will become dangerous through the eyes of some of those around them.

This level of protection does not just involve matters between the police and our sons. This protection encompasses the way the world will constantly overly sexualize our young daughters. Our daughters have been called too grown, too fast, we have been told we are doing too much, for just *being*. Some of our young daughters have been raised without knowing the love of a father, which has inadvertently led to unclear direction when it comes to understanding the role of a man in their life as a husband and partner. Brother, you will be your daughter's first superhero. You will tell her there are no boogie monsters under her bed. At some point, you will put your masculinity aside and have tea parties while she's dressed up as a princess. You will teach her how to use her voice and be assertive. You will tell her she is beautiful. When the world screams at her through their marketing schemes that say she should be a size three with long blonde hair, you will help her understand that her features are a part of her culture, her history, and her original home. Her kinky hair is like the hair of your own mother's. She is a product of you and her melanated skin is absolutely glorious. As a man, you will be equally responsible for building up the confidence of your daughter as her mother will. You will help her understand that her intelligence is her greatest gift, and Black man, you will educate your daughter on the power of discernment. You will raise a Black woman that will be great because of you.

For us as Black parents, these are factors in parenting that we must be aware of early in life. One day your tiny infant will grow, and you will be faced with having heavier conversations with your children than your White counterparts will have to go through. Pregnancy is not the same for us.

Before we can even go into what your partner needs or how you can be supportive, we have to discuss matters of life, confidence, and well-being for our babies. That is what it means to raise a Black son or daughter in this country. You must always be prepared.

# In Care of Your Partner: What Does She Really Need from You during Pregnancy?

Another item Black fathers were concerned about was the care of their partners. What can you do to make your woman feel better during these nine months (technically ten) of gestation?

In Chapter Seven of this book, we discuss hormones. My main advice would be to read that chapter. I would like to advise you to read the entire book, but that chapter is of great importance. During pregnancy, your partner will experience a surge of hormones, mainly estrogen and progesterone, that will cause her to experience symptoms of nausea, exhaustion, and emotions that range from happy to sad, as well as the occasional outburst of tears. Not to mention, her body is changing week by week. Even though we know it is just pregnancy weight, it is weight, and that is a hard pill to swallow. So, what can you do?

## Making Her Feel Sexy Got You into This Position— Don't Forget to Make Her Feel Desired during Her Pregnancy Too

Can you guess how you both came to be expecting parents? A little sexy time, maybe light libations and a lapse in judgment led you to picking up that pregnancy test a few weeks later. Before the baby, your partner probably felt like her sexiest self, especially since she most likely became pregnant during the peak of her ovulation. With the rush of hormones and her growing body, that feeling of loving her physical appearance can be tough to come by. Make sure to still tell your partner how beautiful she is to you. Also understand that you still need to show that you desire her sexually—even if she's not feeling so sexual these days. Intimacy is a communication between lovers, so use your words and express. Light candles over dinner and rub her feet. Kiss her belly and still kiss her nipples. Pregnant women still want to be loved on too. But remember, a pregnant woman's sex drive may not be at its peak. Practice patience with her and try to avoid the guilt trip when she's just not in the mood.

## Show Genuine Interest in All This "Baby Stuff"

As we have mentioned several times throughout the book, women process parenthood by doing all of this preparation. We read the books and blogs, have baby showers, and pre-shop for adorable little clothes. We will talk later in this chapter about how participating in some of these activities can help you get ready for fatherhood too, but it is also a way to bond closer with your partner. She will appreciate your interest, and as a result, will feel closer to you because of your vulnerable efforts.

## Just Be There and Offer Your Support

The best advice that I can offer is to just be there. Learn that being a listening ear does not mean that we are looking for a solution. Listen to your partner and ask her what she needs. Communication will be your biggest ally during this time. There are going to be some gross things that happen during pregnancy. Once I threw up in a cup over dinner. I have upchucked in the car, on the carpet, and even during sex. It was not planned, and it did not make me feel good, but my partner did not judge me or make me feel worse...even if he was silently cursing me out in his head the time I puked in his Benz. He understood that this was something that could not be controlled, and I was doing the best that I could at the time. Back rubs, belly rubs, and foot rubs will get you far. Cleaning the house and unexpectedly coming home with food will get you even further. Afternoon walks and fresh flowers are always appreciated. Better yet, communicate with your partner to find out her exact needs.

Now, what about you? What do you feel that you need?

# Congrats! We Are Expecting!: An Emotional Look into Accepting Fatherhood

Can you take a moment to remember what feeling came over you when the news was shared that you were going to be a father? Perhaps you and your partner have been preparing for this and you were right there when she took the pregnancy test. Or maybe this was truly a surprise and you had to wrap your mind around the idea of fatherhood. If you are a millennial, your freedom may have flashed before your eyes as you wondered, "What on earth am I getting myself into?" However, you have arrived at this point, you are here now and that should be celebrated. Parenthood is not just about Mom and neither is pregnancy. It is important to emotionally grasp that this is your pregnancy too, and just like Mom, you have nine months to prepare for the birth of your baby.

We are all familiar with the science of becoming pregnant: The sperm implants itself into the egg and voila! A baby is born. It is a little more complicated than that (refer back to Chapter One for more info) but the main point is that it takes two to arrive at conception. Instead of saying, "My partner is expecting," try verbalizing, "We are expecting." How does that feel? Even though you may not go through extreme body changes, some men experience couvade, or sympathy pregnancy. If you are feeling moodier than usual, experiencing nausea, weight gain, and food cravings, do not be surprised! Your body is responding to your partner's pregnancy. Those mood swings can make you more irritable, less patient, and give you feelings of confusion. This is why learning to accept fatherhood from an emotional standpoint is extremely important.

Are you freaking out a bit? That is okay. It is also normal, but you should have someone to talk to about it. A lot of our brothers are raised to believe that, as a man, you are supposed to be strong and hold it all in. Don't show emotion. Thankfully, we are breaking generational curses and are learning how necessary it is for our Black men to speak up and speak out. Learning to process your emotions and communicate with your partner or even a therapist is crucial right now. If you have fears around what kind of parent you will be, whether you can adequately take care of a baby, or if this is going to completely change your social life, these are all understandable worries.

It may be time to tap into that brotherhood circle. If you are the only friend in your group that is a father, look on social media and find meetups in your areas. Find men that look like you that can help guide you through this pregnancy journey. The truth is, your partner should be the person you can talk to, but there are things she may not be able to understand. You need a man to speak to. If it is your own father, even better.

# Stay Involved during the Pregnancy

It can seem easy to leave the pregnancy business to your partner, since she is the one carrying the load, but learning to share some of the weight will not only help your partner but also aid you in preparation as well. Take the time to attend prenatal appointments and ask lots of questions. There is no such thing as a silly question when it comes to pregnancy. Pick up a few books that focus on parenthood from a man's point of view or download an audiobook.

Baby showers can seem like a silly idea, but it is one way that women mentally (and financially) prepare for the upcoming birth. Consider having your own or being a part of your partner's shower. Go back to Chapter Twelve to read about baby showers and how they work. While you are glancing back in the book, stop by Chapter Three and learn about how becoming an advocate for your partner during childbirth can save her life.

Next time you are in Target, stop in the baby section and grab a few items that catch your eye. Daddy, you are allowed to be excited. You are allowed to nest as well. Helping your partner pick out items for the nursery, clothing, and car essentials is a surefire way to prepare for pregnancy.

# Creating a Routine That Works for Both You and Your Partner

The best part of pregnancy is that it gives you nine months to create new habits and properly prepare for the birth of your baby. You are not expected to be perfect at parenting, but we know, like anything else, if you prepare even on the smallest scale, you will be further along than if you didn't prepare at all. I am sure I have said it earlier in this book, but do not expect perfection in parenthood. None of us get through it as perfect parents. We just do the best that we can.

One important area of focus that should be considered is a routine for you and your partner. Even though you cannot plan for every single thing, you can check with your job about paternity leave. Only about 13 percent of US workers have access to paid family leave. However, some employers do offer dads time off for the birth of their children. Many men may feel pressured to not take time off from work either because of financial responsibilities or it being unconventional for a man to take paternity leave, but let's take into consideration a nation like Iceland, where 96 percent of fathers take up to ninety days of paid family leave. Countries that tend to embrace the idea of paternity leave tend to produce fathers that are more active and involved as parents.

If you are unable to take paternity leave from work, creating a schedule in the first few months can allow for your partner to feel more comfortable with not having to take on all the responsibility of raising a newborn. You can make suggestions, such as offering her two hours a day for naptime or quiet time if your schedule allows. Create arrangements for who is responsible for dinner on what days. It is also important to consider your own well-being. Do you normally go to the gym every day after work? Discuss why keeping that part of your routine is necessary for your mental wellness or how it can be adjusted to better fit your expanding family.

If you are a smoker and are planning to quit before your baby arrives, creating a routine around your plan is important here too. Can you plan a timeline for an end date and commit to it before baby arrives? If you don't plan to quit, do you have a designated smoking area outside of your home? Can you create one? When planning your routine, just remember that it is okay to make change. Your baby will not be on a schedule immediately, but at least putting one in place can help Mom and Dad handle the transition into parenthood with ease.

. . .

Preparing for parenthood requires more than just healthy eating, finances, and understanding the changes your body is going through. It also means dealing with your own internal conflicts and self-wounds. For those of you who may have had difficult relationships with our own parents, hopefully this guidebook is helping you move into starting your family without carrying over the afflictions of your own childhood. Due to the statistics on fatherhood in our community, there are many conversations to be held around wounds we have been left with by absentee fathers. If you are struggling to let go and forgive your own parents' misgivings, seek therapy. Let that trauma go so you can be the best parent you can be. For now, though, let us get back to preparing for the birth of your baby.

## WELCOME TO FATHERHOOD: A LETTER FROM ANTHONY HAMILTON

Hello young father. This is about to be the most beautiful, frightening, and amazing journey that any man could ever embark on. These nine months of creating this life will change you forever. I encourage you to make this connection with your partner, wife, or your coparenting teammate as beautiful as possible. It is not easy carrying a baby and preparing a life for the unknown. A new life is something that will change you in ways you can never imagine, teaching patience, true love, and giving you the ability to sow wisdom in a seed created by two people. There will be times when she will despise you. Times when your smell, touch, and the mere thought of you will throw her into hormonal overload. Stay the course and it will be different.

Each month there will be a new revelation and a deeper insight she may discover about her body. Things she may love, like her breasts and butt getting bigger! Then there is the reality of, "Oh no! My nose is spreading, and I can't fit anything!" In her eyes, this may all be your fault. Some of these times may be quite hilarious, and other times you will want to pack a bag a leave. *Don't!* Stay there and find ways to make each stage comfortable for her.

You may realize that you are napping and eating more. As men, we tend to gain weight with the mother. That's her fault! The first three to four months are the most stressful and delicate of child development. Try and keep it peaceful and beautiful as much as possible.

Intimacy is key. It is completely safe to continue to have healthy sex. You want to ensure the baby is growing in a safe and healthy energy environment. Make sure she eats healthy foods and drinks lots of water. Hydration is so important. As men we are to pray over them and offer as much support as we can. I can't lie. You may go through periods where you feel you're not ready, and moments of wishing you could change that night. Times when this real-ass future becomes overwhelming. The financial stress of caring for a child or family can be a lot. Take this time to plan, save, and work as much as possible. Stay ahead of the curve and get supplies you may need. Communication is so important.

It helps to keep the peace and give her moments when she feels she's the only thing that matters. The later months of pregnancy will have another set of challenges, each one you will master together. The later months you kind of start to realize it's too far gone to do anything but be prepared. In months eight and nine, the baby could be due at any moment. Make sure to communicate with the doctor and stay on those dates. For me, the night and morning before the labor of one of my children I was a ball of nerves. It took some deep breathing to bring me to. Don't worry. Stay calm. Your sleep-deprived life has just started. Going into labor will be so much to take in and so much to see. Try to mentally be there and experience this miracle with an open heart, mind, and soul. When this baby starts to make way, Mother Nature does a superb job. It is the start of a new life added. Through the blood, mucus, and water break comes your new bundle of joy. It is officially time. Father up and love every minute of it. I enjoyed it so much. I now have six sons. Enjoy young kings. Be fruitful and multiply. Stay the course. God will bless you and enrich your lives.

**Anthony Hamilton**

Grammy Award-winning singer, songwriter, producer, actor, author, and father.

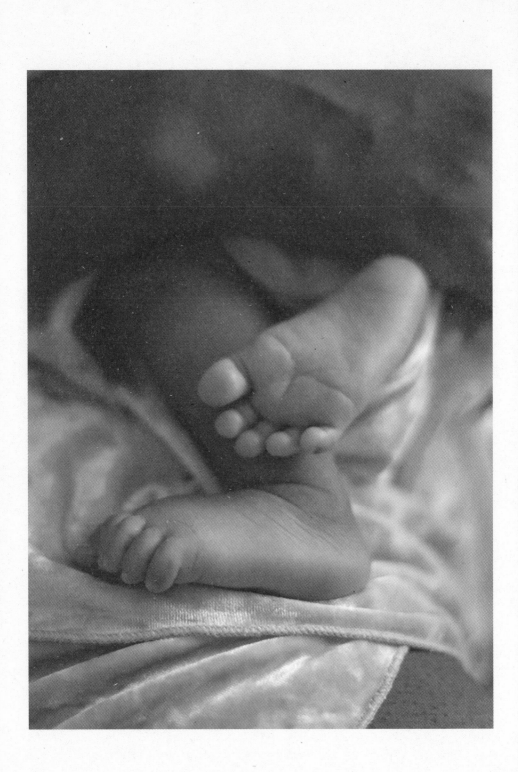

## Chapter Fifteen

# Who Is Braxton Hicks and Why Is My Crotch on Fire?

*Speak up for yourself and what you believe in. You can still be an elegant woman and be strong and powerful.*

—**Misty Copeland**

**No matter how you have** planned on birthing your baby—whether you are having a scheduled Cesarean, a medicated birth, or an unmedicated birth—you will most likely experience some pre-labor symptoms. This part of pregnancy is what I like to refer to as "Shit Gets Real," otherwise known as SGR. You realize that in just a few weeks, you will be coming home with your new baby...one way or the other. As silly as this may sound, my SGR moment did not hit until it was time for me to push. I somehow made it through pre-labor symptoms, my actual labor, and telling the nurse that I needed cocaine to make the pain stop before I was blinded with the fact that I had to push my baby out of my vagina. Everything in the room magically ceased moving, as did the pain of my contractions, and it was as if my OB was speaking to me in slow motion. There was a halo of light around her as she said, "Shanicia, it is time to push."

I want to make you aware of two points: 1) I have never done cocaine and technically, this would probably not be my drug of choice to get through labor. 2) You can do this. You can push this baby out. Do not let my experience completely freak you out. I survived and would gladly do it again under the right circumstances. When I speak about childbirth, especially here in this guidebook, my goal is to always talk to you as your homegirl would. I am going to be painfully honest so that you are not being set up with the okey-doke when it comes to childbirth. Does it hurt? Yes. Will you be able to handle the pain? Maybe. If not, there are drugs for that. No, those drugs do not include cocaine.

# Mentally Preparing Your Mind for Labor

Labor requires a combination of mental and physical preparation. Your labor experience starts in your mind. Leading up to delivery, your body will begin preparing for birth and you will experience different feelings, like Braxton Hicks contractions, Lightning Crotch, mild labor pains, and pressure on your lower belly due to your baby dropping deeper into your birth canal. You may be unusually exhausted, and walking can become even more intense. In preparing your mind for labor, accept that birth is going to happen and empower yourself by having gentle and positive talks with yourself in the mirror. This would be a great time to review your birth plan, look at your baby shower photos, and walk around your newly decorated baby's room to remind yourself that this is all worth it. Stay away from unwanted advice and scary stories of labor—my sincere apologies if you freaked out over mine a few paragraphs back. I am just loving you like your grandmother. A little tough love does the body good.

In all seriousness though, Sis, the first thing you must do in preparing for labor is ready your mind. Even for my sisters who are planning a Cesarean, you must prepare your mind. Here are a few affirmations that you can use for yourself. Stand in front of the mirror every morning and evening before bed and tell yourself:

- My mind is strong.
- My body is strong.
- I am a creator of life.

- There is no wrong way to bring life into this world.

- I am prepared to birth my baby.

- I will manifest a calm and peaceful birth.

Using your words, hearing yourself speak, and guiding your mind to a place of positivity will help to greatly reduce the jitters you may feel leading up to your birth. Another way to prepare your mind is to gear yourself up for what birth is actually like. If this is your first child, you may have never seen an actual birth, and the assumptions in our minds can vary compared to what birth is really like. While you do not want to look up images and videos that will scare you, you do want to set realistic expectations for the process. If you have been attending birth classes online or in person, your teacher, doula, or midwife has probably already had this conversation with you. There are also YouTube videos and Instagram accounts that depict real live birth stories so that you can witness an actual birth.

Fun story: I operate as a womanhood photographer in my free time and photographed my first birth a few years ago. The mother was a surrogate and birthed twins! As a mother myself, it was a completely different experience being on the other side of the table and witnessing her give birth versus being the one going through the process. It felt like I was watching a miracle happen. Women, we are so powerful.

# The Difference between Lightning & Lightning Crotch

If you have made it this far in our guidebook and you are in the last few weeks of your pregnancy, chances are you have already discovered what "Lightning Crotch" is. Lightning Crotch is exactly what it sounds like—a very intense bolt of pain that shoots through your vagina, rectum, or pelvic region. If you are unfamiliar with contraction pain, it is easy to assume that Lightening Crotch is what contractions will feel like, but it is not. This pain can be caused by "lightning," which is your baby "dropping" or changing position to deepen the placement of its head in your birth canal. As your baby's head starts to nest itself into your pelvic bone, you can feel sharp shooting pains. This pain does not mean that baby is ready to come earthside, as you can feel Lightning Crotch weeks before labor actually happens.

Due to the new positioning of your baby, you will most likely experience cramps and lower back pain. This is where your waddle may come into full effect! Your cervix is dilating, which contributes to the cramps and may remind you of menstrual cramping. This can result in your joints feeling loosened, especially in your pelvic region. A hormone known as relaxin works to soften your ligaments to open your pelvic region for the big event.

# Am I Turned on or Is There a Leak "Down There"?

Before having my water break, I assumed that it would be this big ceremonious show like what we see in movies. I would get super worked up about something, maybe an argument or laughing with my girlfriends, and then BOOM! My water would break. I would be whisked away to the hospital and experience this super clean but sweaty birth. There would be exactly four beads of sweat that trickled from my forehead, and I would be full of smiles and tears as I looked down at my beautiful baby.

The truth is that labor doesn't always occur this way. In fact, for some women, their water starts to leak a few weeks or a few days or even twenty-four hours prior to labor beginning. For others, their water does pop, or break, and labor starts. It is different for every mom. Amniotic fluid is the liquid that drains from the amniotic sac. Amniotic fluid is so important because it transfers the nutrients and water between mother and baby and forms the protective liquid that acts as a cushion for your growing baby. If your water breaks too soon and labor has not started, your OB or midwife may suggest labor induction to speed up the birth process. Low amniotic fluid, also known as oligohydramnios, can be easily detected by your doctor. Your doctor may recommend you take bed rest, increase fluid intake, and possibly arrange a Cesarean section.

What the movies do not tend to show us is the "show" that happens before our waters break. The medical term for this is operculum, also known as your mucus plug. Your mucus plug is like the bath stopper to your cervix that keeps your baby healthy by preventing infection. Imagine runny egg whites. While some women lose their mucus plug all at once, right before labor begins, other mothers discard their mucus plug over time and may not even notice the small pieces of mucus that are expelled from the vagina. The "show" looks like a bit of mucus mixed with a bit of blood. The blood should not be too abundant or it may indicate a more serious problem and you should contact your doctor immediately. Once you lose your mucus plug, your body is almost ready for labor. Your cervix will start to soften and prepare for dilation.

If you find yourself on the side of pre-labor when your water is not breaking or leaking, your OB may suggest stripping your membranes, also known as a membrane sweep. A membrane sweep typically happens when you are near your due date or have gone past it. It involves your doctor taking gloved fingers and wiping between the membranes in your amniotic sac in your uterus. Think of it as a really intense internal massage. It should not hurt but may be a bit uncomfortable. Membrane stripping is a natural way to induce labor, and if your body is responsive it can jump-start labor to happen within a few days of your sweep.

## Who in the Heck Is Braxton Hicks?

I have always found it funny that false contractions are named after a man. That is a story for another day. Braxton Hicks are false labor pains that occur before real labor starts. "Braxton Hicks" received its name from the English physician John Braxton Hicks, who discovered them in 1872. I assume he could not think of a better name, so he named the literal pain in a woman's womb after himself.

Braxton Hicks contractions are your body's way of preparing for real labor pains. They feel like a mild tightening of your belly and then a release. Your body is contracting and then letting go. Unlike real contractions, Braxton Hicks contractions typically do not hurt, nor are they consistent. These false labor pains are sometimes triggered by dehydration but can also be caused by heavy lifting, nausea, fetal movement, or sex. While some women experience Braxton Hicks contractions, others do not.

# Pull My Finger

Here is something you may have noticed early during your pregnancy—the inability to hold your flatulence. As you near the time of actual delivery, the difficulty of not farting turns into a difficulty not passing a bowel movement. Is this not a nightmare that every woman considers before labor? No one wants to poo in a room full of doctors, nurses, and their partner. Most especially, none of us look forward to taking a dump on our newborn baby. Once again, our bodies show us how sensitive they can be to the science of birth. One of the signs that labor is near is your body's "emptying" itself out. That's right. At the beginning of labor, most women experience massive diarrhea, which is your body's way of removing fecal matter in preparation for using all of your muscles to push for your baby's arrival.

It used to be required that women fast during the laboring process. It seems logical to blame it on the poo, but food was not suggested because if a woman had to receive anesthesia, she could experience aspiration, which is the inhalation of food or liquid into the lungs. Instead of food, women were given ice chips and water to snack on during childbirth. Imagine the exhaustion! In more recent years, some doctors have agreed that light foods during labor are completely safe. After all, you are performing an Olympic sport. Hydration and nutrition are important. Some food and drink suggestions for labor are Jell-O, popsicles, broths, and juices. Before deciding if food is safe for you to eat during your labor process, please speak with your medical provider.

## This Exhaustion May Feel like the First Trimester

Do you remember how exhausted you felt in the first trimester? Some of that fatigue may be coming back for round two. Your body's preparation for the birth of your baby is hard work and there are a lot of moving parts involved in making sure it all goes smoothly. Changes in your sleep pattern, sleep deprivation, and the return of morning sickness can all be signs that your labor is nearing. You may notice the urge to nap more in the daytime and find yourself fully awake at night. Some of this can be attributed to nerves and to your hormones. Rest as much as you can. These are your final weeks of rest before you find yourself on the full schedule of your newborn.

## A Real Black Girl Moment—Preparing Your Hair for Labor & Delivery

You see, Sis, it was necessary for *The Ultimate Guide to Black Pregnancy and Childbirth* to be written because who else would tell you to get your edges in order before going into labor? Labor is sweaty. Labor is long. Labor will take you all the way outside of yourself. The last thing you want to be worried about is your hair. Our hair is wonderfully versatile, so there are 101 ways you can get your hair done to prep for birth. The goal is to have a hairstyle prior to labor that can last at least two weeks after birth. Let's look at a few go-to protective styles to be considered.

## Two-Strand Twists

Two-strand twists can be a great protective style for birth depending on your hair type and the size of your twists. If your hair type is in the 1–3B hair texture range, you may not consider two-strand twists to be a good protective style for labor, especially if done chunky. The amount of sweat will cause your hair to frizz up and come loose. If your hair is in the 3C to 4C hair texture range, two-strand twists could be a good solution. If your twists are done small, they will hold better and can be worn for at least a few weeks after birth.

## Braids or Twists with Extensions

Braids or twists with extensions are also a good solution for a labor hairstyle. When getting extensions put in, make sure the hair is not done too tight. Tight braids and twists can cause painful headaches, and the last feeling you want to experience during labor is a sore head due to your braids snatching your edges. You may also want to stay away from braids to the scalp that go straight down your back and which cannot be tied up into a bun. If you are laying on your back, it may cause irritation to lay on your hair too. Micro braids, Senegalese twists, or box braids could be better solutions than cornrows.

## Wigs

Wearing a wig during labor can be a great solution, but can also be hot, depending on what kind of wig you are wearing. This serves well as a protective style too, because your hair underneath will be braided flat to your head and can remain that way for a few weeks after birth. The best part about a wig is the versatility to switch up your look whenever you feel like it. You can go into your labor with a short pixie cut and come out with Beyoncé hair. It is completely up to you, Sis.

## Rock Your Natural

Let's be extremely clear: these earlier options are in no way intended to persuade you that rocking your natural tresses during labor is not appropriate. If you wear a fro on a regular basis or would like to do a twist out, this is a great idea as well. For my natural sisters who spritz a little water, pick, and go, keep doing what you do best. Natural is always in.

. . .

Are you feeling a bit more prepared now that you know the signs of labor? On *Black Moms Blog*, I spoke with forty women about what they wish they would have known before having a baby. Some of the responses are funny. Some are practical. Some of the responses are much needed truths. Mostly, I want to help you to find a bit of laughter and excitement in the upcoming birth of your baby and give you space to make new memories all on your own. Here's to "Forty Things Women Wish They Would Have Known before Childbirth!"

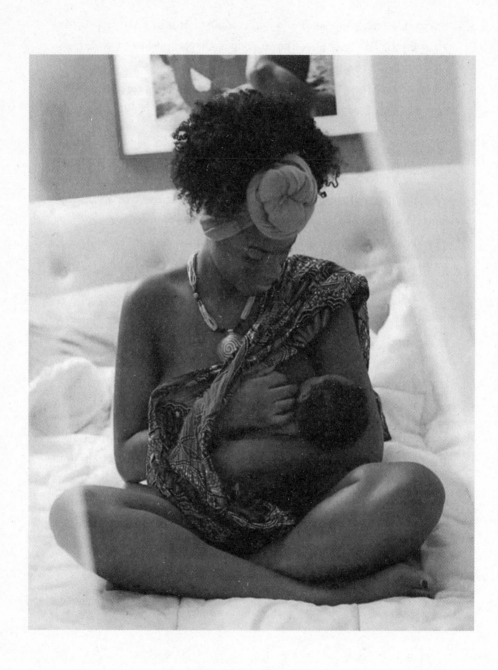

## Chapter Sixteen

# Forty Things Women Wish They Would Have Known before Childbirth

*What you know today can affect what you do tomorrow. But what you know today cannot affect what you did yesterday.*

—Condoleezza Rice

**From the moment we find** out that we are going to
be mothers, we start our long list of dos and don'ts for our
motherhood process. Most of us realize very quickly that nearly
all of our unbreakable rules are breakable; there will be times
when we allow our children to watch television, and every now
and again, it is perfectly okay to eat snacks before breakfast.
On *Black Moms Blog*'s Instagram page, I asked my community
members what things they wished someone would have told them
before they decided to become mothers. Here are some of my
favorite responses:

# Forty Things Women Wish They Would Have Known before Childbirth

1. *"The baby needs nothing but plain white onesies at first. Put the rest in a savings account."* @rawbeauty

2. *"I wish someone had told me you may be in shock the first few days and weeks and may not be 'in love' with your experience or your baby like they said you would."* @carefullycreatedchaos

3. *"Breastfeeding is one hell of a job emotionally and physically."* @kifayate

4. *"It's going to hurt to poop after giving birth vaginally because EVERYTHING gets squashed down there."* @ms.frisco

5. *"You can't do it all."* @code_name_mama

6. *"Trust your instinct, only you know what is best for your baby."* @clau757

7. *"Newborn phase is the easiest part and to thoroughly enjoy it."* @brepoe519

8. *"Your milk doesn't always come in right away and breastfeeding isn't something you or your baby will just know how to do out the gate. YOU WILL STRUGGLE."* @getoutthebox

9. *"That it is okay to not know what you're doing."* @rai.mamas

10. *"It's okay to respectfully decline unsolicited advice, family included! What works for everyone may not work for you."* @bunniebunnybonniebawnie

11. *"Not everything will come "naturally"...it will take real work and perseverance to get through those early infant days. Be kind to YOURSELF! You WILL get there."* @10deroni_

12. *"Take tons of video and pictures because the days will pass fast and you will need something to look back on. You'll realize you've made it so far with your new joy."* @blessedbeyondanything

13. *"Practice encouragement vs. praise. It makes a huge difference in your child's motivation."* @m.joy_xo

14. *"Never compare parenting styles and children's growth. Each kid is different."* @precious.me2

15. *"Take care of yourself! Don't forget you have needs too."* @kokoa_kure

16. *"Relax. Your hormones play a big part in how you feel, so don't sweat the small stuff."* @crossyourheartlove

17. *"Hold your baby as much as you want. One day they will grow up and out of your arms..."* @korien

18. *"Postpartum is real and you don't have to go through it alone."* @abeyoutifullife

19. *"You may lose a nipple once they start teething."* @libertybelle215

20. *"That potty training will require patience like no other, but there is light at the end of the tunnel."* @sharondashariee

21. *"You don't have to do it the way your mom did."* @cristallinay

22. *"Recovery takes longer than six weeks."* @qdpeterson

23. *"Parenthood is YOUR journey. Stop letting family, friends, society, etc. guilt trip you in 'what you should've did.' When I want your opinion, I will give it to you."* @kasualvibes

24. *"Your way is exactly what your baby needs. Trust your instincts and lean in on your better half. He wants to do the best for you as well."* @2blesdchick

25. *"Enjoy your baby. Don't worry about the house...just enjoy."* @mrsjaelynnbell

26. *"Read parenting books now. Take the classes. Hire a doula. Don't go to the hospital alone no matter what. Write a birth plan. Interview doctors. Eat better. Visit more than one hospital. Meal prep your food."* @onlyblackstasinthesky

27. *"Use a backpack instead of a diaper bag. They hold a lot more and have side pockets for bottles and leave your hands free for holding that baby."* @lauramcbroom

28. *"You deserve self-care, give yourself credit, don't lose yourself, it is okay to say not today, get sexy every now and again, you baby won't love you less because you took a mini vacation."* @layla_12_mc

29. *"It's okay to not be okay...and sleep when the baby sleeps. Everything will fall into place."* @hell0_brklynn

30. *"Listen to your body and don't be afraid to ask for help. It doesn't make you weak or less of a new mom learning how to be a mom. And also, postpartum depression is REAL. Talk to your physician about it on checkups."* @mrs.jessicabyrd

31. *"Take more pictures WITH your child."* @punnylady338

32. *"Some days you will have great days and then those days when the baby cries you will sit down and cry too. Have five people you can call anytime and get a break to breathe and relax."* @chandra850

33. *"Sleep will become a luxury."* @crown_meeee

34. *"Don't worry about the baby weight, just be healthy and enjoy your baby."* @mscaribella

35. *"It is okay to not know what to do."* @justrenee00

36. *"Babies cry. Some more than others. They sometimes cry for no reason. The witching hour is real."* @selfexplantori

37. *"Don't feel guilty taking care of you...be a little selfish sometimes. If you good, your baby will be good."* @katcooper516

38. *"That men get postpartum depression too."* @2put_in_motion

39. *"Pelvic floor exercises are important and help you. Later progress on to yoni egg. Trust me!"* @mberry_lish

40. *"At some point, that baby will fall on the floor—whether you drop him/her or they roll off of something, it will happen and you are still a good mom!"* @loulnlco

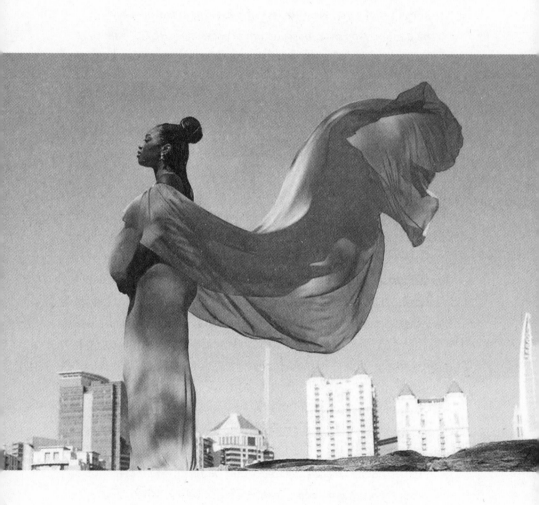

# Chapter Seventeen

# D-Day

*You wanna fly, you got to give up the sh\*t
that weighs you down.*

—Toni Morrison

**I want you to close** your eyes for a moment. Travel back with me, to precisely nine months ago, and remember the feeling you had when those two lines appeared. Or the digitized word *"pregnant"* popped up if you had the fancy test. Or to when your doctor came into the room to announce you were now with child. Or for my super intuitive mamas, back to when you just *knew* you were pregnant. Look how far you have come, Sis. We are finally here.

I reminisce on my own day of discovery from this very moment, as I work from bed with my daughter lying next to me, back to nearly eight years prior to this day when I woke up one morning and knew that my daughter would be in my arms before I closed my eyes to fully rest again that evening. I was in labor and I knew she was coming. I was going to be a mother. It does not matter if this is your first child or your seventh, the moment of birth will always feel like something I can only describe as supernatural. Maybe for women it is the day we discover that we truly are made in God's image. We create life, birth life, and guide that life through the rest of their own lives. It is one of the most fascinating roles on this planet to be a mother. Your due date, as intended by your baby, is your day of arrival to motherhood.

It is nearly impossible to write this chapter with any sort of certainty, as birth will vary from mother to mother. Even for the same mother, each of her births will be different. Some births will be completely textbook from beginning to end. Baby arrives on its intended due date. Labor happens. Water breaks. Baby comes. Other birth stories may include a due date that comes and goes, a labor that lasts for two days, and an unexpected Cesarean. I do not tell you this to put any level of fear in your heart but to help you now begin to unmarry from any idea you have in your head of how your birth story may go. The ultimate goal in childbirth is to have a healthy baby, regardless of the method of delivery. You are a mother if you have a baby by natural birth. You are a mother if you decide to have an epidural. You are a mother if you have a Cesarean section.

As the author of your guidebook and a self-proclaimed pioneer of Black motherhood and mama self-care, I proudly welcome you into our super exclusive club of motherhood. We are honored to receive you, love you, and be of assistance to you during this time. Remember that in motherhood you should never be alone. It is important, truly important, to preface this chapter this way. Before we fully dive into what to expect with delivery, it is necessary to start with self-affirmation. You did this, Sis. Do you feel anxious? Are you calm? Perhaps you're wondering what your delivery will actually be like? Preparation is a solid way to arrive at parenthood, so let's try to cover as much as we can on what to expect on your delivery date.

# Your Body Knows Baby Is Coming before You Do

Your labor is broken down into three different stages. Let's explore each part of your laboring process.

## Stage One: Early/Active Labor

Your first stage of labor consists of two parts. It is divided up into early labor and active labor. It is also probably the part of labor you are most familiar with or what comes to mind when you think of labor. Early labor will most likely be the easiest in relation to pain. One of the first signs of early labor is that your body will release a bowel movement. I couldn't think of a more direct way of telling you this, but you may release waste and it may be a lot. We discussed this briefly earlier in the book so do not be surprised now, Sis. Releasing fecal matter during early labor is your body's way of loosening your muscles for birth and clearing out your bowels to allow for your uterus to contract properly after the baby arrives. Your stool is loosened and released, caused by the release of the hormones prostaglandins. Prostaglandins play a major role in early labor by ripening or thinning out the cervix in preparation for contractions. The technical term for your cervix thinning is "effacement." If the body is not producing enough natural prostaglandins, this hormone may be injected by a doctor to induce labor. We already discussed what to look for in early labor, so if you need a refresher here, go back a few chapters. You may experience some lower back pain, a mild headache and/ or heartburn. If you think you are in labor, use a stopwatch to time your contractions. In early labor, your contractions will be around fifteen to twenty minutes apart and can last from sixty to ninety seconds.

During the stage of early labor, it is best to stay home and relax. At the onset of early labor, you may want to go to the hospital right away, but if you labor is too early, chances are the doctors will send you back home. The labor rule of thumb is if your contractions are five minutes apart and lasting one minute for one hour then you should go to the hospital because you are starting active labor. Remember to speak to your health provider before making any decisions during your pregnancy, including about when it is safe for you to go to the doctor. This rule of thumb is a general statement and should not be considered without consulting your health provider.

In early labor, you can eat light foods. Since your body is cleansing, consider eating foods like fruit, toast, and broths. Stay away from food with high fiber, acidic foods and drinks, and meat. Drink as much water as you can. It is easy to become dehydrated during labor. Your body is about to go through a marathon. Early labor can last around fourteen hours on average for your first child.

## Active Labor

Active labor starts once your cervix has dilated, or opened, to six or seven centimeters. In not so technical terms, active labor is when birth starts to get real. Remember your SGR moments? This may be one of them. Your contractions are going to pick up and things can become a bit more painful. You may just start becoming exhausted during active labor. If you are still laboring at home, this is when you want to head to the hospital. Your contractions are now around four or five minutes apart and last around one minute. For some women, their water may break in active labor, while others may not have their water break until it is time to push. Active labor is when you want to put your Lamaze or hypnobirthing classes to work. Your breathing is very important during this time. On average, active labor lasts around three to five hours.

Something to take into consideration, especially if you are having a hospital birth, is that this is everyday work for the staff. There may be a few different people in and out of your room, and your doctor should have prepared you that they may or may not be available for your birth. If they are unavailable, they will send another OB. Your OB will also normally only be there for the actual birth and not the beginning laboring stages. If you are having a water birth, active labor is when you would get into the pool. If you are planning an epidural, active labor is when you would prepare for your tube. Having an epidural also means having a catheter, which is a small draining tube passed into the bladder to help deplete it of urine.

This is a really great stopping place to go back and refer to Chapter Three on Black maternal health. If something feels off, speak up, Sis. If you are uncomfortable, use your voice. Speak to a staff member, your doula, midwife, your partner, or your friend. Do not be afraid to speak up. It is important to have an advocate at your birth. Once you start becoming exhausted, speaking up may not feel so easy and so you need someone with you that can speak up for you if you are unable to. This is your body and your baby. Always remember to use your voice.

## Stage Two: The Birth of Your Baby

Here's some good news, Sis. By the end of your second stage of labor, your baby will be born! Stage two begins when your cervix is dilated, or opened, to ten centimeters. Your baby is ready to move through the birth canal and you will help guide this process by now pushing with your contractions. Even though your contractions are more intense, they are now a few minutes apart instead of every minute or so. This gives you time to catch your breath in between your pushes. It is hard to put a time on how long pushing lasts. For some women, it can last fifteen minutes. For others, it can last a few hours. Whether you have an epidural or not, your health care provider will most likely guide you through your pushing process. An epidural will alleviate the pain, but you will still feel the pressure of pushing. This helps you know how hard or soft you are pushing through your contractions. One of the most memorable parts of the pushing stage of labor will be experiencing the Ring of Fire. Earlier in the book I told you that I screamed so loud I rocked the entire hospital. This was during my Ring-of-Fire moment. The Ring of Fire is when your baby crowns, or when you are able to see the baby's head coming down through the vagina. Your medical provider may allow you to use your fingers to reach down and touch your baby. Sis, this part hurts. Your baby's head and shoulders will be the most difficult part of your pushing process. The good news is, once the shoulders pass, your newborn will normally be birthed with one or two final pushes.

## Stage Three: The Birth of Your Placenta

I made it through my entire pregnancy, birthed my baby, and was sitting there comfortably when I felt this pressure of another contraction wrapping its way around my back. The nurse on duty for my birth told me it was time to push again. I looked at her like she was crazy. "Birth what?" I asked her. Unlike you, I did not fully prepare for my birth this way. I read a lot of different books and never made it past the first few chapters. So, if you have made it this far, imagine that I am giving myself a silent pat on the back. It's nice to meet you here.

As I was saying, in my own ignorance, I had no idea that I had to birth my placenta. Placenta birth is fairly easy, and your uterus pushes it out five to fifteen minutes after your baby is born. Your doctor will push on your abdomen which can help push the placenta forward to birth. It should not be too painful. You just birthed a baby after all. Along with not knowing that this would happen, I also had no idea that I could keep my placenta either. We discussed what you can do with your placenta after birth in Chapter Eight. If you choose to have a lotus birth, your baby will still be attached to the placenta by their umbilical cord. If not, then you or your partner most likely cut the cord in the second stage of labor.

## What to Expect if You Have a Cesarean Section

Did you know that one third of babies are born by Cesarean in the United States? It is way more common than you may have realized. A C-section can be planned or completely unexpected. Either way, here is what you should expect if you have a Cesarean birth. A C-section begins with your doctor administering an epidural or spinal block to numb only the lower half of your body for the pain of surgery. You are completely awake during your birth and can witness what is happening. Once your IV is done correctly, your belly will be washed, shaved if need be, and an antiseptic solution to sterilize the area will be applied. Right above your pubic line, your doctor will make a tiny incision into your belly all the way to your womb. There are three types of incisions made for C-sections:

1. **Low traverse:** a horizontal incision right above the pubic line

2. **Low vertical:** a vertical incision right above the pubic line

3. **Classical incision:** a vertical cut made more in the center of the belly

The most common incision is a low traverse cut. The muscle right above the public line is thinner, which means less bleeding and easy healing with minimal scarring. 95 percent of C-section incisions are made using a low traverse incision. Once your incision has been made, suction will be applied to remove the amniotic fluid from your womb. You may feel some tugging, and soon after your baby will be pulled out gently by your doctor. Because your newborn did not go through the birth canal, there may be excess mucus in their respiratory tract, and you may not hear that first cry immediately. Don't worry! Your doc will suction out the mucus and the cry will follow soon after.

If your C-section is without any complications, your doc may allow immediate skin-to-skin contact after cutting the umbilical cord. Your placenta will then be gently removed through the incision and you will be stitched up. The actual delivery through C-section only lasts around ten minutes. The stitching of your abdomen can last for thirty minutes or longer.

# The Unofficial Fourth Stage: Healing

The "fourth" stage of labor is also known as the healing or recovery time that happens a few hours after your baby is born. Your uterus still contracts in order to shrink back down to its regular size. The contractions are not as intense as they are during the first stages of labor, but they can be uncomfortable. The hospital may offer you Tylenol or Ibuprofen to help with pain.

What does it feel like to give birth after waiting for so long to meet your baby? While you may not experience the "baby blues," the emotional mood swings and overall moodiness that can happen after birth, you may experience chills, tremors, and dizziness. Personally, I had an extreme adrenaline rush. I felt like I could conquer the world. After twenty-four hours of natural birth, I jumped up from my hospital bed thirty minutes after birthing my placenta and was ready to walk around. My nurse promptly guided me to a wheelchair and told me to sit down. Don't be like me. Allow your body to process what it has just done and regulate back to its normal pattern.

During the recovery period of my fourth stage of labor, I discovered that my vagina was on fire. It gave a new definition to the Lightening Crotch we discussed a few chapters back. I guess pushing a baby through a hole that is normally no bigger than a few inches deep and about two inches across will have that kind of effect. This heat is most likely caused by the bruising and swelling that happens during childbirth. Your OB may give you an ice pack to place in your underwear after birth. Your vagina will be so hot, you probably won't even be able to feel the ice pack. Every dirty rap song I can think of about hot vaginas just came to my head. If only they knew what happens after birth.

# What Happens Next?

## Baby Care

You have waited nine months to meet your baby. Skin-to-skin contact after birth is very important. Immediately after your baby is born, your nurse may use a bulb syringe to remove any mucus from your little one's throat. This is also when you will hear the first cry if your baby was born silent. If there are no complications, you should be given your baby immediately in order to breastfeed. We will talk about breastfeeding in the next chapter. Some new parents opt out of having their newborns cleaned right away and prefer to leave the vernix caseosa intact. The vernix caseosa is the white, cheese-like protective layer that covers your baby's skin after birth. This substance forms in the womb and is thought to have protective components even after your baby is born. The nurses will clean your baby, but after this cleaning it is not recommended that you give your baby a full bath until the umbilical cord falls off and the belly button is healed. Please check with your medical provider for information on when to bathe your baby.

## What Should You Do With Your Baby's Cord Blood?

When your baby is born, there is extra blood that is left over in the umbilical cord and placenta once the umbilical cord is cut. This blood is super rich in antibodies, hematopoietic stem cells, white and red blood cells, plasma, and platelets that can be used to heal diseases and viruses we suffer from. Since the 1980s, doctors have been saving the cord blood from newborns as a way to treat these illnesses. Cord blood can be used to treat more than eighty different types of diseases[6]. By donating your baby's cord blood, you could be an integral part in research that can help find the cures to autism, Parkinson's disease, cerebral palsy, and

6    https://www.whattoexpect.com/pregnancy/cord-blood/what-is-cord-blood-banking/

heart birth defects. You can also save the cord blood for your own child for future use, if they should ever need it.

If you do decide to donate or keep your cord blood, after birth you will be asked where you would like to store your baby's blood—either in a private bank or a public bank. What's the difference? A public cord blood bank is essentially a donation. You are signing away all rights to the cord blood and it can be used in whichever way the cord bank sees fit, for whomever they see fit. This process is free but, as a parent, you are signing away your rights to the cord blood. If you choose to use a private cord bank, you are storing the blood for your own personal use and the blood cannot be used at the discretion of the blood bank. Private cord blood banking can range between $1,300 and $2,500.

## To Circumcise or Not to Circumcise

If you have birthed a son, you may be deciding if you should circumcise or not. Circumcision is when the foreskin covering the head of the penis is surgically removed. Two thirds of male births in the United States are circumcised. Circumcision is believed to have originated in East Africa as a means of purification in order to reduce sexual desire and the urge for pleasure—as it was seen as a dirty behavior to be sexual.

The foreskin is composed of two parts: the outer foreskin, which protects the penis, and the inner foreskin, which is a mucous membrane containing the most nerves and blood vessels. Think of the texture of the inside of your mouth. Between both layers of the inner and outer layer of the foreskin is the ridged band which has specialized nerve endings. When the penis is circumcised to remove the foreskin, a thicker protective skin grows over the penis, ultimately reducing sensitivity. Removal of the foreskin is accompanied by the loss of male secretion called smegma. Men who are uncircumcised can experience similar levels of arousal as the female clitoris and can also produce lubrication when turned on.

America is the only country that practices circumcision for nonreligious or noncultural reasons.[7] Even though circumcision reduces the risk of a baby getting a urinary tract infection, this is only by 1 percent, and circumcised men are three times more likely to experience erectile dysfunction during their more mature years of life. Does this conversation feel a bit one sided? That is not the purpose, but you should be armed with the facts before making a full decision. There aren't many medical reasons for circumcision. One medical reason includes the foreskin being too tight to be retracted over the penis, which your doctor would determine at the time of birth. Another nonmedical reason is that it is deemed more socially acceptable and hygienic to circumcise, and if your son's father is circumcised, he may be more inclined to have his son circumcised as well. Circumcision in the United States has dropped by 55.4 percent, according to the CDC.[8]

Each family must decide what is best for their baby and the decision is up to you and your partner. If you do decide to go the route of circumcision, most doctors will recommend that your baby is circumcised within the first few weeks of life, and if born at a hospital, your son will most likely be snipped within forty-eight hours of birth. The entire procedure only takes around five to twenty minutes, and thankfully, your baby will not be traumatized by the experience. Your doctor will administer a

---

7    thenurturingroot.com/facts-about-foreskin-circumcision.

8    www.cdc.gov/nchs/data/hestat/circumcision_2013/circumcision_2013. htm.

topical anesthetic or a nerve blocking anesthetic by injection at the base of the penis to perform the circumcision. Your newborn may also be given a pacifier dipped in sugar water known as a sucrose pacifier, which can reduce any stress or anxiety in your little one.

A circumcision can be performed by three different methods: with a Mogen clamp, a Gomco clamp, or by the Plastibell technique. The Mogen and Gomco clamp methods both include using a probe to separate the foreskin, the blood flow is then reduced by a clamp and the foreskin is removed with a scalpel. The Plastibell technique also uses a probe to separate the foreskin from the penis, but instead uses a plastic bell which is placed under the foreskin, and a suture is placed around the foreskin to restrict blood flow. After a week or two, the foreskin will fall off on its own. With the Mogen and Gomco clamp methods, your doctor will rub a petroleum ointment over the penis and wrap it to keep any irritation from happening with the diaper. With the Plastibell technique, there isn't any wrapping required. Your newborn will experience a bit of soreness, but there shouldn't be much bleeding at all, and the penis will heal fairly quickly—around seven to ten days.

## Your Care: The Fire Crotch

Your "down there" will need some extra love and attention for the next few days. You will most likely be given an ice pack to reduce the swelling and bruising. Birth gives an entirely new meaning to "beat it up." I laugh a bit at how vulgar men can be when it comes to making love to a woman and to our literal life source. The vagina is magical. You won't look at rap lyrics the same ever again after having a baby.

Your perineum will need to be cleaned with warm water, either with a bottle after you pee or in the shower or bath. Most hospitals provide you with a little spray bottle to gently cleanse your perineum after birth. You do not need to rub it or touch it at all. If you have any tears, your stitches will absorb within seven to ten days of application. Be gentle with your lady parts. If you feel comfortable, start light Kegels to regain strength in your vaginal muscles. Refer back to Chapter Eight to read about perineum care and Kegels. Don't worry, Sis, your vagina will snap back just fine.

Remember that annoying peeing sensation you had during pregnancy? It is suddenly eradicated once delivery is over. Using the bathroom still becomes a major accomplishment after birth, and your doctors are going to want you to do it fairly quickly. This just ensures that everything is back to normal after your baby is born. You will probably be able to pee right away, but having a bowel movement may take a little more time and effort. Most women are able to "do the doo" two to three days after baby is born. Some doctors do prefer to know that you have passed at least one bowel movement before discharging you from the hospital. Your muscles just went through a lot and your mind is probably psyching you out as well. If you are struggling to use the bathroom, try eating foods with heavy fiber content and drink lots of liquids. You can also take a light stool softener to get things moving.

Here is another surprising fact that I did not discover until the day of delivery: you are going to bleed. A lot. It is almost as if your body has been saving up all of your missed period blood for this very moment. Afterbirth bleeding is called Lochia, which is the bloody discharge of tissue, mucus, and blood from your uterus. Lochia lasts roughly around two to six weeks after birth and passes in three stages. The first stage is called Lochia rubra. Lochia rubra is dark red and lasts two to four days after birth. The hospital will provide you with the largest pads you have ever seen in your life, or with pregnancy underwear to catch your Lochia rubra. Regular pads won't cut it. You want to change your pads every four hours at minimum to reduce the risk of an infection. Lochia serosa is the second stage of afterbirth bleeding, and it is pinkish brown and lasts from around four to ten days. With Lochia serosa, you can start using a regular pad. Lochia alba is the last stage and lasts anywhere from ten to twenty-eight days after birth. This afterbirth blood is a whitish-yellow color. Lochia should not smell much different than normal menstrual discharge. If you notice a foul odor, consult your doctor immediately.

## C-Section Care

Official C-section care instructions will be provided by your doctor. Make sure you ask any and all questions about how to handle your aftercare. You will be sore after birth and your abdominal area will be tender. Do not try to be Superwoman during this time. Allow those around you to help you and help with your newborn. After your C-section, your doctors will encourage you to walk after about twelve to twenty-four hours. This helps prevent blood clots, constipation, and reduce gas buildup in your stomach. Your rest is important. It will allow your body to heal normally. You should walk every day, shower normally, and be gentle with the abdominal area—especially with laughing or coughing. On average, women recover from a C-section within four to six weeks.

## Bain: A Haitian Afterbirth Bath

In Haitian culture, women are initiated into motherhood with a series of three baths, known as "bain" baths, during their postpartum period, which lasts for forty days. It is not strongly recommended to soak in a bathtub after birth, so rather, in Haitian culture, the woman sits over a large pot or tub of very hot water to wash and pour water over herself, normally with the assistance of an elder, doula, or midwife. The new mother is to stay home to rest, heal, and limit her interactions with the outside world as much as possible. These baths are prepared with herbs, sunlight, and fruits. The first bath is made from a combination of:

- Papaya
- Sour orange
- Soursop
- Mint
- Anise
- Bugleweed
- Eucalyptus

This bath causes the muscles to contract after birth. The mother is rubbed with herbs and heavily "massaged" by an elder. I use quotations around massage because if you know, then you know. It's more of a loving beating than a massage. The pressure of the massage helps to relax the body but also tightens the muscles. A special tea is made from the same herbal blend for the mother to consume as well.

The second bath takes place three days after the first bath and lasts for three days in fortified water that is warmed by the sun. The final bath, the third, happens exactly one month after birth and is a cold bath. This is the final step in tightening the muscles and the bones. During this postpartum period, the mother's stomach is bound tightly to put the body "back together." The heated steam from the bain bath is meant to draw out any tissue that has been left inside the mother after birth.

This healing method is also practiced in Jamaica, but the postpartum period of bathing normally lasts for nine days with one bath each day. These are cultural practices passed down generationally, but the use of herbs, yoni steams, and afterbirth bathing rituals has become more widely accepted in the Western world.

## Belly Binding: Should You Do It?

Postpartum belly binding is the tradition of having a long cloth wrapped around your abdomen area, from your rib cage down to your hips, intricately tied to support your abdominal muscles after childbirth. Belly binding, or bengkung, originated centuries ago in Malaysian culture. It has been practiced traditionally across Asia, Europe, and Latin American, and has just recently, in the last few decades, become a sensation in the United States and other countries. Belly binding is believed to help remove extra fluids after birth, shift organs back to their original position, provide back support, and close your hip joints.

Culturally, belly binding is referred to by different names but provides the same benefits. Asian mothers refer to the cloth as a "sarashi" and use it to tighten loose skin and retone the abdominal muscles. In Hispanic cultures, the cloth is referred to as a "faja." Belly binding can be an intricate process with very specific knots tied around the abdomen and adjusted as your uterus and your stomach reduce in size, or it can be an overall wrapping of the belly tied in one single knot. For full effectiveness, belly binding is recommended immediately after birth and has to be worn for a minimum of forty days. Please consult with a professional before proceeding.

If the traditional form of belly binding is not your forte, there are modern alternative wraps and corsets that you can use as well. Depending on your insurance, the cost of your wrap may be fully or partially covered.

## What Is Diastasis Recti?

Diastasis recti is when your abdominal muscles, or your "six pack" muscles, separate after birth. Do not freak out, Mama. It is more common than you think and happens to more than 60 percent of birthing mothers. Diastasis recti can occur from intense strain on the inner abdominal muscles, and with pregnancy your relaxin and estrogen hormones are working overtime to make sure your stomach properly stretches to accommodate your growing womb. Women who have multiple births back-to-back (think Irish twins), are pregnant with high-birth-weight babies, or are over thirty-five are more prone to Diastasis recti. Symptoms can include bloating, constipation, and lower back pain. To do a self-check, you can lie on your back in a sit-up position and raise up in a half sit-up with one hand supporting your head. With your other hand, feel in between your abdominal muscles to see if there is a one to two finger gap. If there is a gap, you may have Diastasis recti. While standing, if you notice a bulge or pooch that makes you still look pregnant after delivery, this is also an indicator of Diastasis recti. Make sure you check with your medical provider for an accurate diagnosis.

## How to Treat Diastasis Recti

Belly binding or wrapping is a good way to treat Diastasis recti. For more extreme cases, physical therapy can also be recommended. Some light ways you can self-treat Diastasis recti at home include always being aware of your posture, avoiding lifting heavy objects, being mindful of how you are lifting yourself up either to get off of the floor or in and out of bed, and using a pillow to support your lower back. If you notice that your Diastasis recti has not healed on its own after eight weeks postpartum, you can begin practicing these exercises as well as using Kegel exercises to strengthen your pelvic floor and core muscle exercises for your ab strength. Consult your doctor before beginning any workout routines that you do not normally practice.

# Another Conversation on Black Maternal Health

Chapter Three of our guidebook is most likely one of the most important chapters you will read. I encourage you to reread it in full several times during your pregnancy and before you go into labor. To reiterate, Black maternal health refers to the dedication to educate about and to reduce the Black maternal mortality rate during and after childbirth. Black Maternal Health Week, founded by the Black Mamas Matter Alliance, is held during the week of April 11th to the 17th. Per the website, BlackMamasMatter.org, Black Maternal Health Week is meant to:

- Deepen the national conversation about Black maternal health in the United States
- Amplify community-driven policy, research, and care solutions
- Center the voices of Black mamas, women, families, and stakeholders
- Provide a national platform for Black-led entities and efforts in maternal health, birth, and reproductive justice
- Enhance community organizing on Black maternal health

Creating websites, movements, books, and summits to discuss keeping Black women alive during the birthing process is not something that we want to do. It should not have to happen. This work is necessary and requires your participation. This work needs you to use your voice. We need you to speak up. As you experience your own delivery day, do not hesitate to scream, shout, and demand attention if you feel anything that feels like too much. Say something if it feels like too little. Speak if you have a feeling of dread in the pit of your stomach. Do not let up. It can save your life. We have heard too many devastating accounts of Black women who have died during childbirth. Black women like Sha-Asia Washington and Yolanda "Shiphrah" Kadmia. Celebrities such as Beyoncé and Serena Williams have publicly spoken out about the hardships they faced while birthing their children. I implore you to always use your voice.

Now that we are nearing the ending of this book, I want to leave you with a few chapters of information discussing breastfeeding, postpartum, and getting your groove back after becoming a mother.

## Chapter Eighteen

# A Conversation with Krystal Milky Mama Founder, Krystal Duhaney

*Dreams are lovely. But they are just dreams. Fleeting, ephemeral, pretty. But dreams do not come true just because you dream them. It's hard work that makes things happen. It's hard work that creates change.*

—**Shonda Rhimes**

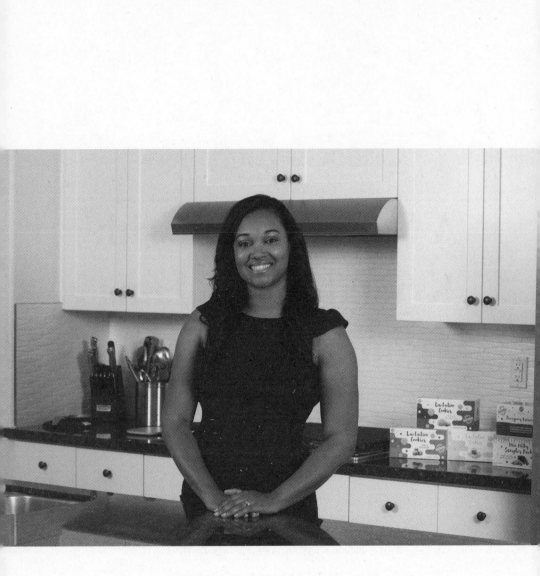

**Milky Mama was created by** Krystal Nicole Duhaney, a registered nurse, international board-certified lactation consultant, and breastfeeding mommy of two. After having her second child and returning to work, Krystal struggled with her milk supply and realized that there were very few resources for breastfeeding mothers in the same predicament. She knew then that she had to come up with a solution that would help to increase her milk supply. Using her knowledge as a registered nurse and her love for baking, Duhaney developed a milk-making cookie recipe and fell in love with the results. These lactation cookies dramatically increased her supply. Soon after, she decided that she could not keep her discovery a secret and had to share this with other mothers who were going through a similar situation. In November of 2015, Milky Mama was born.

Today, Milky Mama's product line includes delicious Lactation Cookies, Brownies (which are Krystal's favorite), Emergency Brownies, Tropical Iced Tea, Lactation LeMOOnade, Lactation Smoothie Mix, and Herbal Supplements.

Along with offering tasty treats and beverages, Milky Mama has also generated a following among women who help support each other and other women on their journey. "It was also important for me to create a village of support, because I needed it and I craved it. Having the extra support is so vital. It is heartwarming and a huge passion of mine to give breastfeeding support. I receive so many responses from customers sharing their experiences: because they eat my treats, they are going strong with lactation. It's so amazing what a little extra support can do." Milky Mama facilitates weekly Facebook chats and a lactation support group.

Whether you're a first-time mother or a Hollywood celebrity, Milky Mama can empower you with the physical and emotional support you need to raise happy and healthy babies!

# A Conversation with Krystal Duhaney

**Tell us a little about your work and how you specifically help Black mothers.**

**Krystal Duhaney:** Milky Mama provides an unparalleled sisterhood of support that prenatal and postpartum parents need. With online breastfeeding courses, a support group with over 25,000 moms, virtual lactation consultations, weekly Q&A sessions with a lactation consultant, and effective lactation supplements, Milky Mama provides a full-circle experience that improves the health and wellness of both mom and baby. Committed to eliminating the racial disparities experienced by Black breastfeeding parents, Milky Mama launched a Lactation Consultant Scholarship Program to help certify Black lactation consultants.

**What are myths around breastfeeding? Are there any that are specific to our community?**

**KD:** Here are some common myths regarding breastfeeding:

- **Myth:** Breastfeeding is supposed to hurt, and your nipples are supposed to crack and bleed in the early weeks.

**Fact:** While nipple tenderness and soreness are normal, severe pain, cracking, and bleeding are not and are usually the sign of a shallow latch or ill-fitting flange.

- **Myth:** The larger your breasts, the more milk you'll make.

**Fact:** Breast size has nothing to do with your ability to produce milk. The ducts and glands in your breasts, not the fatty tissue, help facilitate milk production and breastfeeding. So, whether you're an A cup or a DDD, you can produce plenty of milk for your baby.

- **Myth:** You should not breastfeed if you are sick.

**Fact:** In most cases, you should continue to nurse even if you are sick. When you are sick, your body produces vital antibodies to help prevent your baby from getting sick or to help lessen the intensity of your baby's illness if they do happen to get sick. Of course, be sure to perform proper hand hygiene and wear a mask if you have a contagious respiratory illness such as the flu, a cold, or COVID-19.

- **Myth:** Black women don't breastfeed.

**Fact:** Although Black women have the lowest breastfeeding rates compared to any other race, we *do* breastfeed, and the number of new breastfeeding mothers is increasing every year! Causes like Black Breastfeeding Week help to educate and empower Black women to breastfeed proudly and confidently, despite the multiple racial disparities that we experience.

**What at-home methods do you recommend to a mother who desires to be a better breastfeeder?**

> **KD:** If you're having trouble, reach out to a lactation consultant. They can assist you in person and virtually to help troubleshoot your breastfeeding issues. I'd also recommend joining Facebook groups dedicated to breastfeeding and lactation. These groups allow you to connect with fellow nursing and pumping parents (and sometimes lactation consultants) to provide support. Additionally, if you are unable to connect with a lactation consultant, things like breastfeeding videos, YouTube videos demonstrating latching techniques and other breastfeeding tips, and educational websites such as Kellymom.com can be great resources.

**Do supplements really work? What are their benefits? Can you name a few go-to supplements that you recommend?**

> **KD:** There are many foods and herbs that have been known to help increase and promote milk production. However, it's important to know that there is no supplement in the world that can ever replace frequent and effective milk removal. If you aren't removing milk from your breasts (either by nursing or expressing milk) frequently throughout the day, your supply will likely decrease. Things like oats, flax seeds, brewer's yeast, moringa, goat's rue, and more are common galactagogues that help promote lactation.

**A lot of Black moms now are first-generation breastfeeders. What advice would you give to a mother who may not have the best support system at home for breastfeeding?**

**KD:** Oftentimes, Black moms experience a lack of breastfeeding support from their friends and family due to a lack of education regarding the benefits of breastfeeding. It may help to educate your family and friends about the many benefits of breastfeeding so that they can be part of your support system. If you still are lacking support at home after educating your family, it can be very helpful to join a breastfeeding support group specifically for Black breastfeeding mothers. Studies show that mothers who have a support system are more successful at breastfeeding. Build your support system however you can.

### Does pumping still make you a breastfeeding mom?

**KD:** Absolutely!! The definition of breastfeeding is the action of feeding a baby with milk from the breast. If you're feeding your baby breast milk or donor milk, no matter how much or how little, you are a breastfeeding mom! It's important to realize that every breastfeeding journey is different and beautiful in its own way. Appreciate and celebrate your unique journey and avoid comparing yours to anyone else's.

### What advice do you have for a new mother when it comes to breastfeeding?

The best thing you can do is to educate yourself and build your support network. Research shows that when you have adequate support and are well educated regarding breastfeeding, you'll have a more successful breastfeeding journey. Taking a breastfeeding course, finding a lactation consultant to refer to, educating your family and friends, and connecting with other breastfeeding/pumping mothers are great ways to set yourself up for success.

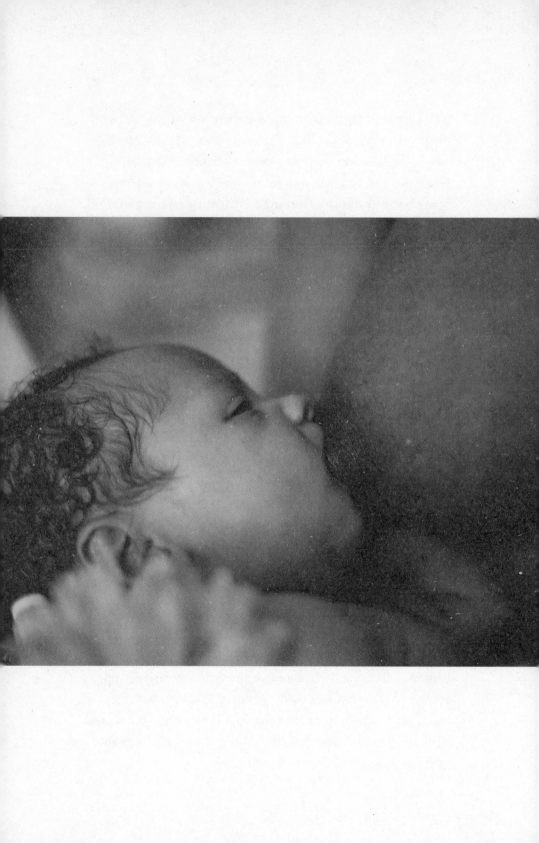

## Chapter Nineteen

# Breastfeeding and the Black Mother

*Beauty is not just a White girl.*
*It's so many different flavors and shades.*

—**Queen Latifah**

**I remember being pregnant with** my daughter and one of the elders in my community, an older Black woman that had birthed her own tribe of children, told me that in order to prepare for breastfeeding I should take a toothbrush and brush my nipples in the shower. She told me that this would harden the skin on my nipples because the suction of the baby would be "uncomfortable." Looking back, I realized that she was being polite in saying "uncomfortable." My first few weeks of breastfeeding were a much more intense experience.

One night, I sat on the sofa crying silently between my mother and my daughter's father. Tears spilled over my cheeks as we watched a movie, and I held my newborn daughter. I was three days postpartum and my breasts were painfully engorged with milk. The only way I can describe how milk engorgement feels is to compare it to what I would assume breast implants feel like right after surgery. My breasts were at least two cup sizes larger than normal, they were extremely hard, and I felt this low vibrational pain that would migrate around my chest. My nipples were chafed and calloused. Even though my daughter had a decent latch, she would suckle, rest for only a moment, and then cry. I felt as if I were not providing her with enough milk and was somehow starving my child. How was this happening? I had survived med-free labor and delivery. This was supposed to be the easy part. I always remember this day. I was a first-generation breastfeeder.

That day and many other days, I sat between people I loved the most and felt completely alone and isolated. My partner could not help me with breastfeeding because he was a man who had no experience around breastfeeding. My mother could not help me because she had not breastfed me or my brother. My friends could not help me because I was the only one in my friendship circle that had a baby. Like many Black millennial women, I was embarking on this journey alone. As I began to educate myself on breastfeeding and provide breastfeeding support to mothers through *Black Moms Blog*, I learned there was so much more to explore with Black breastfeeding that went far beyond the feeling of your nipples when your newborn feeds. I also realized that breastfeeding was not something that I witnessed growing up. I never saw my aunties do it or any other Black woman for that matter. Breastfeeding was not a conversation topic at all. As the question of *why* began to rise, looking into the history of breastfeeding in the Black community helped me to understand a deep generational curse.

# A History of Breastfeeding in the Black Community

Without the proper resources, my breastfeeding journey only lasted six months. I felt defeated. In fact, the statistics show that Black women are less likely to start breastfeeding than mothers of any other race, and even less likely to continue breastfeeding for six months.[9] Only 69 percent of Black women initiate breastfeeding compared to 85 percent of White women.[10] The question that is often asked after hearing these statistics is: Why? There are many reasons. There are unfortunate events deeply connected to our race as a people: a history of wet nursing,

---

9    www.cdc.gov/mmwr/volumes/68/wr/mm6834a3.htm.

10    www.pbs.org/newshour/health/racial-disparities-persist-for-breastfeeding-moms-heres-why#:~:text=Overall%2C%2083%20percent%20of%20U.S.,same%E2%80%93a%2016%20percent%20disparity.

the oversexualization of our bodies, and a lack of economic and familial support are just a few.

Cultural reference should always be considered when discussing breastfeeding. During slavery, Black women were used as wet nurses.[11] A wet nurse is someone who breastfeeds another woman's child. The true definition of a wet nurse uses the word "employed," but replace that word with "forced" and the reality becomes clear. It is generational that Black women have developed a disdain for breastfeeding due to our historical relationship with wet nursing. Because of wet nursing, many Black women were unable to breastfeed their own children. Can you imagine the psychological effect that must have in a moment that every mother should enjoy?

Economics should also be considered. Comparing single family households, 65 percent of Black children are raised in single-parent households, while 24 percent of White children are. Black mothers are overwhelmingly the breadwinners of their families. They are more than twice as likely as White mothers and more than 50 percent more likely than Hispanic mothers to bring in the main source of income even when partnered or married according to the Center for American Progress.[12] Because of this, Black women are more likely to return to work sooner and formula feed their newborns instead of breastfeeding.

Black women have a history of adverse health outcomes that are significantly reduced by breastfeeding. Breastfeeding lowers the risk of obesity, osteoporosis, and breast cancer, and reduces

---

11    muse.jhu.edu/article/647289.

12    www.americanprogress.org/issues/women/reports/2019/05/10/469739/breadwinning-mothers-continue-u-s-norm/

the risk of type 2 diabetes by nearly one half if done for more than two months.[13] African Americans are 60 percent more likely to be diagnosed with diabetes than non-Hispanic Whites.[14] Breastfeeding can help lower the risk of obesity, osteoporosis, and breast cancer, which Black women die from at the highest rate.

I realize that this may all feel a bit heavy. You are currently pregnant, trying to become pregnant, or have just birthed your baby. The last thing you want to hear about are more statistics telling Black women that we are just not getting it together like we should. It is important to understand the history though. By understanding the history we erase the ignorance, and in this case, erasing the ignorance can improve life not only for us but for our babies and the future generations that come after us. If breastfeeding has ever made you uncomfortable, you are not alone. Sometimes it is important to just know that one truth—you do not have to do this by yourself.

# Are You Feeding Your Baby Enough?

One of the biggest stressors new moms experience with breastfeeding is this overwhelming fear that you are not feeding your baby enough. What is worse than thinking that you are

13   www.nih.gov/news-events/nih-research-matters/ breastfeeding-may-help-prevent-type-2-diabetes-after-gestational-diabetes#:~:text=Breastfeeding%20for%20longer%20than%202,by%20 more%20than%20one%20half.

14   minorityhealth.hhs.gov/omh/browse. aspx?lvl=4&lvlid=18#:~:text=African%20American%20adults%20are%20 60,compared%20to%20non%2DHispanic%20whites.

starving your child? Here is a hint: there are not many other things. To first understand what is "enough," we must educate ourselves about the size of your baby's stomach and the simple fact that sometimes babies just cry. It does not automatically mean that you are not breastfeeding your baby enough milk.

Newborns have very small bellies. Think glass marble small. Overfeeding your baby in the first few days can actually do more harm than good. Too much milk can cause stress on a newborn's kidneys. In the first few days of breastfeeding, you will produce a thicker, more yellow breast milk called colostrum. Colostrum is important because it is full of protein and nutrients, and it is exactly what your newborn needs in their first days of life. Colostrum helps fight infection, build the immune system, support gut function, and reduce jaundice—which is when your baby is born with a yellow tint to their skin and eyes. Jaundice is not just discoloration. It occurs when the liver is not properly breaking down the red blood cells. Jaundice is fairly normal in newborns and will clear up on its own. Your hospital or birthing center may speed the process along by placing your newborn under a phototherapy light known as a bili light. The light gets its name from bilirubin, which is the yellow substance that causes jaundice.

Your body knows what it is doing in the first few days when it comes to milk production. Your milk comes in three different stages. The first is colostrum. The second stage is transitional milk. This milk is slightly orange because it is a mixture of your colostrum and your mature milk. Your transitional milk comes in three to five days after birth. Your mature breast milk comes in a week or two after birth and is thinner and white, even though it can appear to have a bluish tint at first. In a typical birth, you will produce the right amount of milk in the beginning stages to feed your baby. Your newborn's first bowel movements will be influenced by colostrum. It works almost as a mild laxative that helps move meconium, which is a black and sticky tar like substance that happens as a bowel movement. Let's take a moment to discuss bowel movements and how they relate to breastfeeding. Also, for my mothers who are formula feeding, it is important to understand what is considered "normal" when it comes to passing waste in the first few days of life. Depending on whether you are breastfeeding or formula feeding, bowel movements can vary in color and texture. Whether you breastfeed or formula feed, your baby will produce and pass meconium within twenty-four to forty-eight hours of birth. Around day four, the meconium will turn a greenish-yellow color. For breastfed babies, the greenish-yellow bowel movements will most likely remain the same color. Your baby will pass bowel movements on average three times a day but can also have as many as twelve! Do not be alarmed if you are changing diapers a bit more than expected. This may only last for a few days and then your newborn may only have a bowel movement once every few days. For formula-fed newborns, the greenish-yellow waste will turn light brown or green and you can expect around one to four bowel movements every day. Around the thirty-day mark, your newborn will only pass a bowel movement on average once every other day.

Think of the size of your newborn's belly like this: at one day old, your newborn's belly is the size of a marble. At three days old, your newborn's belly is the size of a ping-pong ball. At ten days old, their stomach has expanded to the size of a large egg. Around your third or fourth day of breastfeeding, you will notice that you begin to produce more breast milk. Are there ways to increase milk production if you feel that your baby is not producing enough milk?

# Dealing with Low Milk Supply

My first bit of advice when it comes to dealing with low milk supply is to speak with a lactation consultant that can better help you. A lactation consultant is a professional who has been trained to aid you in breastfeeding. After birth, your OB or medical provider should recommend a lactation consultant to you. If you are struggling with latch, low breast milk, extremely sore nipples, insufficient weight gain for your newborn, birth of multiples, or if your newborn is special needs, a lactation consultant can help address your concerns and put you on the right track with breastfeeding.

Do not feel guilty or overwhelmed if you assume that you are not producing enough milk. Most women produce more than enough milk for their babies—almost one third more milk! So, if you are feeling that you aren't producing enough, chances are it is probably more mom guilt than truth. Even still, there are real factors that do cause low milk supply. No matter how rare low milk supply is, there are a few reasons why a mother may experience it. Factors such as premature birth, not breastfeeding enough, or waiting too long to start breastfeeding can contribute to low milk supply. Other factors like obesity, high blood pressure, and diabetes can also cause low milk supply. If you would like to produce more breast milk, here are some ways that you can boost milk production:

- Avoid smoking and drinking. Alcohol and nicotine can reduce your milk production.

- Breastfeed immediately and consistently. Practicing skin-to-skin contact can jump-start milk production. As soon as baby is born, begin breastfeeding if you are able. On average, you should breastfeed every two to three hours.

- Practice breastfeeding from both breasts instead of favoring one breast over the other. This can cause milk production to decrease in the breast less used. Do you want lopsided breasts? I think not.

- Be cautious of medications. There will be a warning label on your medications that inform you if your medication is safe to use while breastfeeding. Always check with your medical provider if you are hesitant about any medication you are currently taking.

- Pumping in between breastfeeding can help increase breast milk.

You can also try these foods and herbs:

- Oatmeal
- Fenugreek
- Increased water intake (at least eight glasses a day)
- Yogurt
- Lactation cookies

# The Perfect Latch

Latch is an important topic when it comes to breastfeeding. How your baby latches, or how your baby attaches their mouth to your breast, can make or break your breastfeeding experience. If you notice, I did not state that latching is when your baby only attaches to the nipple. A good latch means your newborn has latched to the entire areola, not just the small nipple of your breast. In pregnancy, you may have noticed that your areolas became larger, darker, and bumpier. You can blame this one on pregnancy hormones. Maybe this is nature helping your baby find your nipple. This has not been proven but it is an assumption often made.

Maintaining a good latch is essential to breastfeeding successfully. How can you promote a good latch? If you plan to introduce pacifiers, wait until around three to four weeks. This will allow your baby to establish a bond with your nipple and not confuse your nipples with other nipples. If you are able, this should also apply to bottles. WIC, a special supplemental nutrition program for women, infants, and children, offers the following suggestions for steps to making a good latch:

- Tickle your baby's lips with your nipple. Doing so will cause the baby to open their mouth wide to suckle your breast for feeding.

- Aim your nipple higher instead of placing your nipple directly into your newborn's mouth. Make sure their chin is not tucked into the chest and their head is angled upwards.

- Your baby's tongue should be extended in preparation for breastfeeding. Help this by aiming your baby's lower lip away from the base of your nipple. Make sure their lips are outward like a fish and not tucked in. Your breast should fill your newborn's mouth as opposed to your baby latching to only the nipple and pinching to suckle breast milk.

Breastfeeding may be a bit uncomfortable at first, but it should not be extremely painful. If you are experiencing any extreme pain, see your medical provider immediately.

# The Benefits of Breastfeeding—for Mom and Baby

Here's some amazing news, Sis—breastfeeding is packed full of benefits for you and baby. I know there is a lot of stigma around breastfeeding in our community, but breastfeeding can help with everything from decreasing your risk of certain diseases to shedding those baby pounds. Breastfeeding is extremely beneficial for your baby as well. Breastfeeding increases nutrition and helps build the immune system in our newborns. Let's look at a few ways breastfeeding is beneficial—for mom and baby.

## For Mom

### Weight Loss

Before I get into this conversation, I just want to let you know that a "snapback" is not real. In a recent conversation with Jet Setting Jasmine, psychotherapist and adult entertainer and educator, she expressed, "I don't believe in a snapback because we can't go back. We are different after each pregnancy and childbirth, so why are we trying to go back? I believe in looking forward. How do I want to show up in the world now?" I felt that. When it comes to talking about weight loss after your baby, we have to get out of the mindset of thinking we are going to look like our favorite influencer who supposedly snaps back three days after giving birth. Something you should know about pregnancy weight loss is that a lot of it is genetics, Mama. If you have a predisposition to be naturally smaller, you will be naturally smaller. If the women in your family tend to be a bit on the thicker side, you may wear those extra pounds a little while longer. Some women gain twenty pounds during pregnancy and others gain thirty pounds. We are all different. Don't forget, that your fave on Instagram posting snapbacks is normally posting photos tilted to an angle, wearing black, and is standing ten feet away from the camera. Every time I see those photos, all I can think is: Sis, you are still bleeding. It is perfectly okay to rest.

Let me also be clear here because I know people...ahem, pregnant mamas can be sensitive. I am not shaming any mother that does snap back and wants to post about it. If that is you, make all the social posts you want. I am specifically speaking to my mothers who leave feeling shitty about themselves after seeing another woman humble brag about how her body went back to "normal." What is normal anyway?

If you are looking for your imaginary snapback, or even better, your snap forward (can we really make this a thing?), breastfeeding is the way to go. According to research, breastfeeding can help you burn an additional five hundred calories a day.[15] Breastfeeding moms are also more aware of what

---

15    www.ncbi.nlm.nih.gov/pmc/articles/PMC5104202/

they are putting into their bodies and are likely to eat healthier because they are feeding their children what they are eating.

## Postpartum Bleeding

In a previous chapter, we discussed Lochia, which is the bloody discharge of tissue, mucus, and blood from your uterus. Because breastfeeding releases oxytocin, nicknamed the love hormone because of all of the warm and fuzzy feelings it gives you, this causes your uterus to contract and expel more blood quicker. In turn, you can have less postpartum blood in the long run, or your postpartum bleeding could end faster than if you chose not to breastfeed at all.

## Lowers the Risk of Serious Disease

One of the best benefits of breastfeeding is that it lowers the overall risk of serious and potentially fatal diseases. Breastfeeding lowers the risk of:

- Breast cancer
- Ovarian cancer
- Diabetes
- Hypertension
- Endometriosis
- Osteoporosis
- Arthritis
- Cardiovascular disease

Given the statistics that show Black women have a higher predisposition toward several of these diseases than our White counterparts, this is reason enough to breastfeed for at least six months. Breastfeeding also helps reduce the risk of less threatening but still serious infections and illnesses such as urinary tract infections and anemia.

## Breastfeeding Benefits Emotional Stability

Remember we talked about all the warm and fuzzy feelings we get during breastfeeding because of oxytocin? It all comes in handy when speaking about emotional stability. In the next chapter we will discuss postpartum depression, but we can jump in gently here. Breastfeeding releases the hormones oxytocin and prolactin, which reduce stress and promote a healthier and more emotionally stable mother. Babies who breastfeed can experience increased calmness and are less fussy, which also brings calmness and peace to mom. There is an increase in bonding time between mom and baby as well.

# For Baby

## Your Breast Milk Is What You Eat

Expectant mamas have a few things in common. One of these is making sure our babies are healthy. Breast milk contains the ideal amount of proteins, vitamins, and fat to keep your baby's immune system at an optimal level of health. Your diet contributes plenty to the nutritional value of your breast milk too. The better you eat, the better the breast milk is that you provide for your child. Your diet also affects how your infant will digest their milk. With breast milk being a lot easier to digest than formula, your baby ends up with less gas and tummy upset.

## The Health Benefits

Children who were breastfed tend to have lower risk of cancers, allergies, eczema, asthma, are less likely to become obese, and have reduced risk of contracting certain viruses. Breastfed babies are three times less likely to have ear infections and five times less likely to contract pneumonia and lower respiratory tract infections. Mothers who breastfeed help boost the immune system of their newborns by passing white blood cells through their breast milk. Vaccinations are a sensitive topic, and whether or not to vaccinate is a personal choice for each family, but breastfeeding is shown to increase the antibody response in babies versus infants that are formula fed. For information on vaccinations, please consult your medical provider.

## Breastfeeding Reduces the Risk of SIDS

In Chapter Eleven, we defined SIDS, or Sudden Infant Death Syndrome, as the sudden, unexplained death of an infant that happens during periods of sleep. According to research done by Pediatrics.org, breastfeeding for as little as two months, even combined with formula feeding, can reduce the risk of SIDS. Breastfeeding between two to four months can decrease SIDS by 40 percent.[16] Breastfeeding for four to six months reduces SIDS by about 60 percent, and breastfeeding longer than six months reduces SIDS by about 64 percent. Exclusive breastfeeding for two to four months reduces SIDS by about 39 percent, and exclusive breastfeeding for four to six months reduces SIDS by

---

16   pediatrics.aappublications.org/content/140/5/e20171324

about 54 percent. Statistics are pulled from a study done by Healthjournalism.org.[17]

Why does breastfeeding scientifically reduce SIDS? We have no exact idea. Scientists have a model known as the "triple risk model" which points to three underlying causes that can increase the likelihood of a baby unfortunately passing away from SIDS. These factors include the vulnerable developmental period in a newborn's life specifically between the ages of two to four months old, environmental triggers such as smoking, and biological, genetic, and neurological disorders which can affect how easily a newborn is prone to waking up. With breastfeeding, babies tend to wake up easier and more frequently than formula-fed babies. Socioeconomic factors also contribute to SIDS and breastfeeding. Lower income and less-educated mothers are less likely to breastfeed, which means that our babies, our Black babies, are twice as likely to die from SIDS than White newborns. Breastfeeding can literally save your baby's life.

Take a deep breath, Sis. The recurring theme of our guidebook is that knowledge is power. These statistics and facts are not presented to scare you but to educate you. The more you know, the more informed decisions you will make throughout your pregnancy and motherhood journey. We now have a wealth of information right at our fingertips and in this guidebook, I am focusing on the information that directly affects our pregnancies, labor, delivery, and the first few months after giving birth. Refer back to Chapter One of your guidebook. My words were this: There will be plenty of books that tell you that your belly has grown to the size of an avocado or a pineapple. We need viable

---

17    healthjournalism.org/core-topic.
php?id=4&page=glossary#casecontrolstudy.

information that truly prepares us for motherhood. We need the information that includes what pregnancy and childbirth is truly like for Black mothers. If we do not look out for each other, who will?

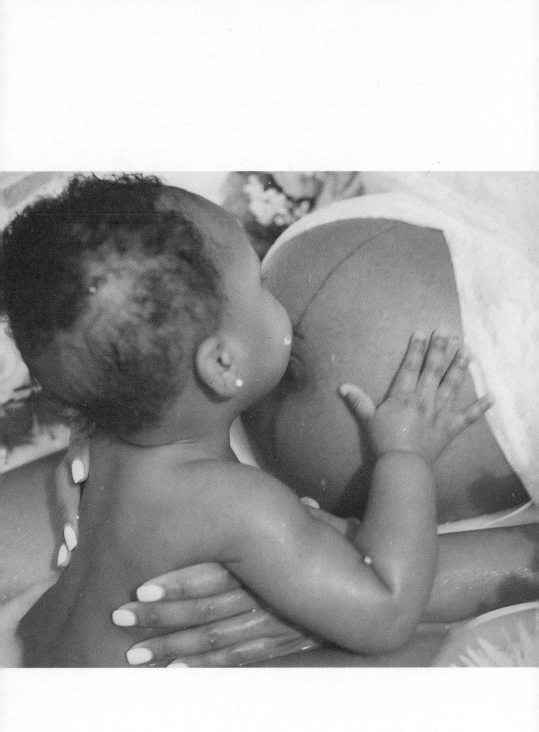

## Chapter Twenty

# Hey Single Mama, You Are Not Alone

*I always believed that when you follow your heart or your gut, when you really follow the things that feel great to you, you can never lose, because settling is the worst feeling in the world.*

——

**—Rihanna**

**We all become pregnant in** different ways. Some women plan for pregnancy with their partners. Others decide a solo birth is a better choice for them and go through sperm banks, insemination, or intentionally make arrangements to become pregnant with another person to coparent. There are moms who have babies through one-night stands, relationships, and with friends with benefits unintentionally. Babies make it into this world through a variety of situations. No woman is better than the next because of how she chooses to give birth. We are all strong for choosing to give birth, no matter the circumstance.

I remember the first time I learned that women choose to have babies without a partner and the first time I met a teen mom who was also married. Both of these occurrences happened in the same summer when I had just turned nineteen years old and finished my first year at Georgia State University. I was determined not to go home for the summer, so I knew that getting a job was my best bet for staying in the city. I also needed my place of employment to pay for my housing, food, and basically my entire life. There was only one position that fit that entire to-do list, and it was becoming an orientation guide leader for my college to give tours to incoming freshmen for the following year. I worked twelve-hour days and even started drinking coffee in the morning. I officially felt like an adult. Even still, there were so many parts of me that were completely ignorant and naive. I did not grow up surrounded by babies. I did not have any real friends who were teen moms, and I did not have younger siblings or cousins running around. The first time I had ever babysat a small child by myself would not happen for another few years after my college epiphany. I freaked out and called his mother to pick him up after he threw up a pink cupcake all over my carpet. I thought I had poisoned the poor child.

My friend and fellow orientation guide leader Ashlyn was a nineteen-year-old, married, and pregnant college student. Ms. Sylvia, the assistant in the office I worked from that summer, was in her late thirties, single, and pregnant. These two drastically different situations seemed like they were on opposite ends of the spectrum. A person may have assumed that Ashlyn's situation should have been Ms. Sylvia's and Ms. Sylvia's life should have been Ashlyn's. Even deeper than that, I realize what a statement our director was making in hiring Ashlyn as a guide leader. I am sure seeing a Black and pregnant teen was off-putting for some parents, but even more it showed real representation, that a woman, no matter her status or what decisions she made for her womb, still had the right to attend college and further her education.

Through the gossipy grapevine of young college students, I learned that Ms. Sylvia had chosen to conceive her baby as a single woman. She was in her late thirties and waiting for Mr. Right to come knock her up was not on her agenda. Looking back, I am aware of how strong she must have been to make a decision like that. She became another Black single baby mama; not because someone left her but because she made a choice for herself. My friend, on the other hand, taught me that all young girls were not just single baby mamas. Ashlyn is still married to this day and her family of three has turned into a family of five.

What about those of us who have become statistics? What about the Black girls and women who are raising babies on their own? While the world is slowly evolving, the stigma of the Black baby mama is still a heavy pill to swallow. 65 percent of Black mothers are single parents versus 24 percent of non-Hispanic White mothers.[18] I will not argue against the fact that children benefit greatly by having two parents, but even more than two parents, children need to be raised in a loving and communicative household and in a positive community overall. Beyond the politics of how many parents a child should have, our focus here is on you, Sis. I am speaking directly to the mama who is embarking on this motherhood journey alone. What are some ways you can still feel supported as you become a solo parent?

# Redefining Your Support System

In Chapter Seven, we discussed how life can drastically change once you become pregnant. Birthing a baby will help you to understand how important a loving support system is for you, your baby, and your mental health. Being the first to become pregnant in my group of friends changed my life in ways I did not fully expect. I have mentioned this earlier in this guidebook, but I will stress it again: becoming a mother in your twenties has become just as taboo as having a baby in high school. By accident, I did not announce on social media that I was pregnant until I was close to six months, and at that point I figured I better say something instead of appearing on Facebook with photos of a newborn. Of course, those close to me knew. The announcement was met with some mixed reviews—mostly congratulatory ones, a few side eye ones, and then of course there were the: "Oh! I just can't wait to meet the baby!" replies. Just a heads up: most of the

18    datacenter.kidscount.org/data/tables/107-children-in-single-parent-families-by-race#detailed/1/any/false/37,871,870,573,869,36,868,867,133,38/10,11,9,12,1,185,13/432,431.

people who say, "Oh! I just can't wait to meet the baby!" never actually meet the baby. Once my daughter was born, it felt as if I had become initiated into some new secret society. I had become a *mother*. Even though I had prepared for this moment for nine months, the beginning stages were like watching my life as a fly on the wall. It was a completely out-of-body experience, and all of the delusions I had of just giving birth and continuing on with my life as if nothing had changed quickly flew out the window.

There is a scene from *Sex in the City* where single mama Miranda has just given birth to Brady. She is struggling to get Brady dressed and prepare herself for work in the morning while Carrie is on the phone ranting about some self-caused small problem in her personal life. Miranda tries to be a good friend and listen but eventually snaps at Carrie, telling her she doesn't have time to listen to her problems because she has a crying infant she needs to worry about.

This.

All the books, all the reading and studying I did to become a mom, did not prepare me for the hard times of adjusting to not only motherhood but to the lack of empathy from those who did not understand what becoming a mother involved. A part of me does not completely blame them because, just like them, I was unprepared too. I was unprepared when my supervisor told me that my staff didn't respect me because I could not go out drinking at the bar after work. When I informed him I couldn't because I had a three-month-old at home, he said, "Just bring the baby." When one of my friends (*mostly the ones who have never met the baby*) would call to invite me to dinner or on a grand shopping trip and I would decline, their response again would be, "Just bring the baby." I was especially unprepared for becoming a single mother when my daughter was just three years old. Becoming a new parent, especially a single mom, is just not that simple. A part of you will want to continue on with your life as is with your current friends. It is difficult wrangling a small child and staying completely engaged in conversation with another adult. It is nearly impossible to enjoy red wine or try on clothes during a girls' shopping day when your infant has pooped all over themselves. If this was your life as a single woman before having children, you may feel this urge for all things to go back to "normal." Then you realize that your life has changed.

There is a reason that moms have other mom friends. Your mom friends will understand that a play date is more than just getting the kids together but also serves as a time for Mom to have a normal conversation with another adult while equally occupying the attention of her child. Mom friends won't look at you crazy when you plop out a boob in the middle of lunch to feed your newborn. When you are a single mom, mom friends understand that you may not have anyone else at home to allow you to nap. So coming over to help out with lunch or laundry every now and again is a necessary part of friendship. Your friends without children can also be a helping hand if they truly understand that your circumstances are different. What about those friends who cannot understand your new life? Learn how to compartmentalize your old friendships. Your old sista friends still have a place in your life, they just may not hold the same capacity as they have in the past. Save those friendships for a fun night out or annual girls' trip. Learn to understand that people can normally only love you through the lens of experiences that they have had themselves. If your friend has never experienced motherhood, then it may be complicated for her to understand just what it is that you need as a mother.

Where can you meet new mom friends? The internet has been a wonderful place to connect with other mothers. Through my platform, *Black Moms Blog*, we strive to connect mothers together from all over the world. Find online communities through social media and become active in them. Join Facebook groups and inquire about mommy meetups in your city. Local libraries and bookstores have story time for children and your local park will normally have a gang of mothers with their strollers and other children. Open up your energy to receive the type of love, friendship, and support you need. This advice is not just for single mothers but new mothers in general.

# Nurturing Your Village: Remembering to Appreciate Our Families

I grew up in a household where we all managed to survive our adolescence without any teenage pregnancies. My brother left at eighteen to join the military and I left at the same age to go off to college. I had one associate who was a teen mom. She lived with her mother, and consequently her mother bore most of the weight when it came to actually raising her child. Her mother would babysit, change diapers, and feed her grandchild when my friend needed some downtime. I also watched this friend berate her mother when her mom would say *no* to watching her son. Being sixteen, I did not understand how selfish my friend was for this. She wanted to go, and her mom was not doing anything. Why wouldn't she just watch her grandchild?

Grandparents are supposed to want to babysit and watch our children. They love them, care for them, and they are supposed to want to help you.

This was my mindset at sixteen. And a part of me took pride in graduating high school and making it through college not having to depend on my parents to take on this task. I told myself, when I became a parent, my husband and I would have sole responsibility for raising our child. In the years before becoming a single mother, this was true. Even still, during my years of being a parent, I have gained a deeper respect for the notion that it takes a village to raise a child.

## We Need Our Families

When I speak of families, I mean blood and extended. In reality, none of us really do it all on our own. Most parents have a friend who will babysit on occasion, we take our children to daycare or school, and grandparents sometimes help on the weekends. There are even babysitters' apps that you can use to call a nanny at the last minute if absolutely necessary. There are many people who assist us in taking care of our children. Because we are the primary parents, we can take it for granted when others help us. We start to feel entitled to this help and somehow make our choice to become parents the weight on someone else's shoulders.

We are no longer polite to the childcare providers: "Of course she better take care of my child. It's her job."

We no longer respect our parent's schedules: "Of course her grandmother does not mind watching her overnight. It is her grandchild."

We no longer see that our friends have their own bag to carry: "Of course she will help me. She sees how hard I am working by myself."

This blind eye that we turn to those around us on account of our own responsibility has to stop. We need our families. We need this help. And no matter how hard it is to see, no one has to help you.

# "No" Does Not Mean I Don't Love You

No means no. That is it. It can reference exhaustion. It could mean the person is unable because of prior obligation. If you find yourself questioning the validity of a friend or family member's care for you based on the one time they answer no to your request for help, it is time to hold up the mirror. Do not become the social media disgruntled person. We all know them. They are the people who surround themselves with the same group of people, and as soon as they are not getting their way, we see posts like this:

"I guess I can only depend on myself."

"I can't depend on others to do for me the way that I do for them."

"Forget everybody. All I got is me."

Newsflash: Yes, you are right. All you do have is yourself. Everything else is a blessing.

Here's the thing, we are responsible for every decision and action we make in this world. If you are a person who is constantly finding themselves on the bad side of the card, then maybe it is time to reshuffle your mental deck. Release the entitlement mindset. Appreciate when someone offers you a helping hand. And most of all, be grateful.

## Take the Time to Say Thank You

How often do you say thank you in your mind but the words never actually leave your mouth? It is the same process as apologizing. Sometimes we say "Thank you" or "I'm sorry" to our loved ones in our minds but fail to tell the person how we feel. A thank you goes a long way. A sincere thank you will increase your chances of receiving help again and can make a person feel appreciated. Never forget how much of an impact your words can have. Once a month, set an intentional timer to say thank you to those who have helped out. You can write them a letter, send a text, or make a phone call. The thank you does not have to be an extremely grand gesture, just a simple acknowledgement of your appreciation for their help.

## Return the Favor

Take a look at your relationships with others. Are they balanced? Do you find yourself asking for help more than participating in the partnership? Are you angered when you do not get the desired result from a person, and does it cause you to withdraw from that relationship until your anger has subsided? If you find yourself on this side of your relationships, you may not be returning the favor. Returning the favor does not always mean doing the exact same thing to help someone as they did for you. Check in with your friends and family. Ask your family, "Am I being needy?" The answer could be a tough pill to swallow but necessary to hear. A needy person never realizes that they are needy. They just live with the idea that everyone else is selfish and they are the ones who are constantly helping others. It is a hard delusion to break. If you find yourself wondering where you fall, start finding ways to return the favor to those that help you. It does not have to be much. Offer to treat them to dinner, give a listening ear in a time of need, or surprise them with money next time they offer to help you. Always ask yourself, "When was the last time I did something nice for this person who is helping me with my heavy load?"

## Appreciate Your Family

This task can be more mental than physical. Release all anger associated with not being helped and getting your way. Hold up the mirror and see yourself and understand this fact: no matter who is behind you, the load is still yours to carry. Do not see your load as a burden but find ways to make it easier and try not to pass it on so much to others. Realize that every helping moment is one to be thankful for, and when those helping moments are few and far between, others simply cannot do it. That is okay. Never get so wrapped up in your own world that you forget that your family has their own responsibilities to attend to. Appreciate them. Love them. Cherish them.

# I Am Not a Single Mama. I Am a Single Woman with a Child

When my daughter was three years old, her father and I decided to separate. At the time, emotions ran high, and the following two years was a whirlwind of relearning how to communicate, coparent, and not constantly fire shots every time one of us became upset with the other. I had become a single mother and it felt like my entire life had been flipped upside down. My anger and bitterness began to not only affect me, but it started to intercede with the relationship I had with my young daughter. She would do a normal agitating four-year-old thing and I would become upset because I was the only parent there to rectify the issue. I was not supposed to be going through this parenthood journey alone. I made sure of that. Her father and I were in love, we were planning to marry and be successful parents. When our outline did not go as planned, my self-awareness kicked in to stop the train wreck of becoming a bitter baby mama. Listen, Sis. When you decide to give birth, your child becomes *your* responsibility. You are allowed to be upset because you did not get whatever fairytale that was fed to you throughout your adolescence, but your reality will still be the same. You are now raising your child alone and you have to not only make the best of your life, you have to *thrive* in your life. Later in this guidebook, we will discuss how to learn to love yourself again. It does not matter if you need this lesson in regaining your self-worth after giving birth or if you need it to heal after a bad breakup, the information will still apply. Let's focus on changing the "single mama" narrative.

Whenever you complete a government application—for your driver's license, voter registration, or even your taxes—there are three little square boxes that give you the option to choose single, married, or widowed. There is another box that asks you to specify which gender you identify as—male or female. Man or woman. With these boxes, the government application declares you a single woman, married woman, or a widowed woman. When we become mothers in failed relationships, we no longer identify as a single woman, we proudly rename ourselves as single mothers. We fought for this title to show strength and that, regardless of our circumstances, we are parenting on our own. There are women for whom the title of single mother really does apply. This chapter is not aimed to detract from any of their hard work. I want you to consider, though, renaming yourself again. I want you to reclaim your single womanhood, not your single motherhood.

In my folded relationship, I gained a wonderful coparent. The road was not easy, and it took much fine-tuning. After years of trying to make something work that didn't, we applied that same energy to parenting our daughter, something that we both loved to do. As my daughter's father stepped into his role as a fully capable parent, I did not feel the urge to become bitter or upset that he had moved on and was happy. I looked at my own life and realized that I was happy too. I had healthy friendships, my business was taking off, and I was learning more about my self-care and how not to place guilt around the things that I loved. The term "single mother" comes with so much heaviness. I wanted to shake off my guilt from becoming single while also ridding myself of the trauma of mom guilt. I decided that instead of being a single mama, I would be a single woman with a child. This new title liberated me. It set me free of the chains of feeling unworthy and eliminated the need to overexplain why I was a single mother. Instead, when I introduced myself as a single woman with a child, my simple statement read like a fact. It was a decision, and I had learned to accept and thrive in its identification. I learned that just because the relationship with my child's father was unsuccessful did not mean that his entire fatherhood could be denounced as nothing. I had become a single woman. My child had not become a single daughter.

Earlier in the chapter, we learned an alarming statistic. 65 percent of Black women are considered single mothers. This is a reality in our community and an ultimate healing has to take place. New parenthood, especially as a Black woman, is a constant readjustment to our mental state. For some women, the transition can be easier than others. How do you determine if the struggle you are feeling is normal sadness or something more? In the final few chapters, we will learn how to identify postpartum depression and how you can learn to get your groove back after having a baby, single or married.

## Chapter Twenty-One

# A Postpartum Conversation with Midwife Aiyana Davison

*When you take care of yourself, you're a better person for others. When you feel good about yourself, you treat others better.*

—**Solange**

**Throughout *Oh Sis, You're Pregnant!*** we have focused on the many changes that occur in our lives, from changing hormones, to changing diapers, to relearning what the word "support" really means. An important topic of new motherhood is the postpartum phase and what may come with that new time in your life—depression. For this topic, it was important to speak with a professional who teaches Black women to recognize what postpartum depression is, how to identify it, and learn to overcome it.

Aiyana Davison (pronouns: she/her/hers) is a certified nurse midwife and women's health nurse practitioner-BC currently practicing in Southern California. As a passionate professional, some of her most pressing priorities include: shedding light on and helping to eradicate the inequalities that exist within health care, addressing the crisis that Black women (people) face in the United States, the provision of quality care for all individuals and families, and the preservation of the legacy of Black midwives and birth work. With this in mind, Aiyana uses her business and social media platforms under the name The Vagina Chronicles (@thevaginachronicles) to educate, engage, and create safe spaces for those interested in all things birth work, empowerment, and overall obstetric and gynecologic health. She encourages healing through sharing and vocalizing stories (as opposed to the long-standing historical traumatic secrecy) to aid with the advancement and success of vulnerable communities.

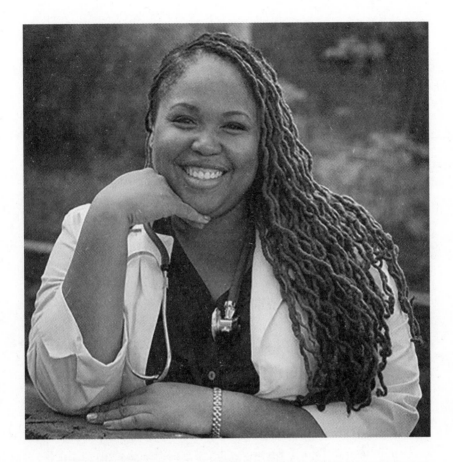

# A Conversation with Midwife Aiyana Davison

**Can you define postpartum depression in your own words?**

**Aiyana Davison:** To understand postpartum depression, it is important to also understand postpartum blues. Postpartum blues is almost like an "expectation" but does not necessarily happen for every birther. Blues is adjustment—hormonal, physical, mental, spiritual, and in role and lifestyle—to having a baby. From mood swings to crying and changes in routine, it can be overwhelming, but the blues also tends to resolve itself within a short period of time. Postpartum depression is different. It is a state, a condition, that spans well past postpartum blues and creeps into nearly every aspect of a person's life after birth. This type of depression can happen as early as one week after a baby has been born and as far out as one year after birth. It is more than feeling overwhelmed, although that can be a part. It can be fueled by fatigue and/or lack of support but also can continue despite adequate rest and help. The classic signs are a disconnect between parent and baby—not bonding, not wanting to take care of one's self or anyone else (other children included), wanting to harm oneself or someone else. Then there are some signs that may go unnoticed because they are not as common or can't be grasped in a postpartum questionnaire. These could be signs like headaches, stomach upset, or back ache. Guilt is another common theme seen during this time. Postpartum depression is a place that many parents do not want to be mentally, but they have difficulty finding ways to free themselves of the emotions and thoughts that weigh them down.

**Tell us a little about what you do and why you work with Black mothers specifically?**

**AD:** I am a certified nurse midwife and I care for a fairly diverse population. As a midwife I provide care to "low-risk" individuals. We say from menarche (the start of periods) to menopause (the cessation of periods) and everything in between and beyond. You can come see me for a Pap smear, pregnancy, for birth control management, abortion care and resources, troubleshooting your period, STD screening, sexual dysfunction, vaginal issues, and so much more.

I love what I do, and I aim to offer the same care to everyone. But I am not ignorant of what my people are going through. Black parents, Black mothers, and children are still dying at alarming rates. What I am passionate about is caring for my people. It's not a question, it's not up for a debate—my people are important to me. Whatever role I can play to prevent, reverse, or stop us from dying, I will. I've watched as my own mother, my aunt, close friends, and family have been disrespected, their concerns invalidated, and symptoms ignored, and it all points to systemic racism. I will go to work for my people because we deserve so much better than what we have been given in this country. In addition, I do this for the legacy of Black midwives. The story of Black midwives as healers is not a myth. It is a true calling, and we are seeing the return of and the visualization of Black midwives as healers and doers of the work needed in the community. I am here to be a part of that and to continue the legacy as well as pave the way for future Black midwives. We need us.

### How are Black women more affected by postpartum depression than our White counterparts?

**AD:** Postpartum depression affects roughly 20 percent of folks who have given birth in general, and those numbers are much higher amongst the Black community. What's vastly different is how it manifests amongst Black people as well as how it is communicated (or not communicated) to providers or even family/support persons. It is one thing to have postpartum depression and to have support and the privilege to speak freely to a therapist, but Black womxn sometimes face the unthinkable when it comes to postpartum care. We battle access to care—rides, distance, childcare, and finances. Then there is the fear that perhaps this will cause someone to take our children away, because we are speaking up about our own needs and somehow this translates to our "inability" to care for our children or ourselves. There is also the stigma within our families and socially that therapy is "not designed for us," so we avoid it for more fear of judgment. Then there's the struggle to be heard by someone who will actually listen to us. The list goes on and on and this has lasting impact on how we heal and cope.

### Is postpartum depression the same as just being sad on any given day?

**AD:** Postpartum depression is more than just being sad on any given day. Yes, that can be a part of it, but as mentioned it often encompasses our whole world. Every day activities are a struggle. At times a parent may seem fully functional but there is a void and darkness that they battle. What's important to note is that because of the resiliency of our people, we often "work through" these feelings. This is not to say that a parent is no longer depressed but that there are so many other elements to everyday life that Black parents may dismiss, feelings and major concerns, in order to keep momentum going at home or, again, in fear of what the repercussions might be.

### Can a mother conquer postpartum depression on her own?

**AD:** Quite simply, no. The work of conquering postpartum depression requires help. This can be the help of a partner, doula, midwife, therapist/social worker, psychiatrist, family, friend, or support group. What I do know is that having a baby and then caring for that child is not a solo journey. It does, sometimes, require us to dig deep and speak up for ourselves to the right people willing to help.

**What are myths around postpartum depression that you work to dispel?**

**AD:** *That having postpartum depression means that your baby will be taken away.* Unfortunately, there are some cases where parents have been reported or threatened with social work cases and/or removal of a child from their custody for conditions that can be treated, but typically this is not the case. A social work referral may, in some instances, provide valuable resources for parents suffering from postpartum depression.

*That postpartum depression is only treatable with medications.* This is simply not true. There are many ways to help treat or cope with postpartum depression. This is why a conversation with a trusted provider as well as your support network is necessary. Also, if there has been any prior history with anxiety, depression, or other mood disorders prior to pregnancy, creating a plan for pregnancy and postpartum can be an invaluable tool for management and preparedness.

*That postpartum depression is easily identifiable.* Actually, some parents are really good at hiding it from their support group, providers, and even themselves. It can be deceiving when they bury themselves in their work or place focus on other aspects of life.

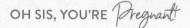
**What advice would you give to a new mother who may be experiencing postpartum depression?**

**AD:** Build your community before having your baby. Plan postpartum meals and help around the house. Choose people who know you and your personality to check in on you and to help. These are the people who may be able to help identify when you are not quite "yourself" and when you may need to consider reaching out for professional help. Sometimes, they may be the ones to reach out for help on your behalf. Find an online or local support group. Use your voice. We have been silent in many arenas for far too long. We must speak up to get the help we need and deserve. Lastly, share your story. If you have experienced postpartum depression or anxiety before and know other parents in your circle, hearing your journey may be the fuel for their journey or give them knowledge and resources they did not know were available.

No matter how dark it may feel at any given moment, you do not have to go through postpartum depression alone. Black women, we pride ourselves on being strong. The one time you do not have to be strong is after childbirth. Lean in on your community. Reach out to family, friends, your doctor, or practitioner, and ask for help, Sis.

# Chapter Twenty-Two

# #THISISPOSTPARTUM: A Chapter on Abortion, Surrogacy, and What Comes Next

*There have been so many people who have said to me, 'You can't do that,' but I've had an innate belief that they were wrong. Be unwavering and relentless in your approach.*

—**Halle Berry**

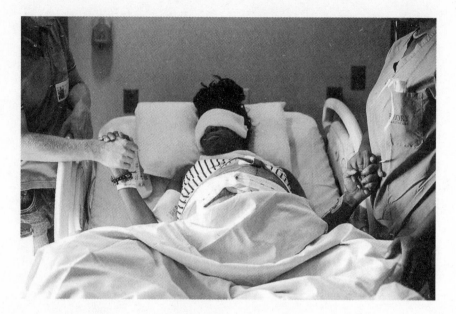

Dr. Vernette rested in her hospital bed, still a little out of it from naturally birthing two babies. Baby A came out headfirst. Baby B was breech.

"How do you feel?" I asked her.

"I feel complete," Dr. Vernette answered simply.

Dr. Vernette is the mother to her own two littles, a practitioner in holistic health, and at that moment, a Black surrogate mother. I recently heard it said Black women don't adopt or become surrogates because we are too busy making our own babies. That may be true, but for Dr. Vernette, there was a much bigger picture.

# The Reality of Abortion

At sixteen years old, Vernette became pregnant. Like most sixteen-year-olds, she was frightened, and under pressure, she made the difficult decision to terminate her pregnancy. In the media, abortion is portrayed as this selfish act that women seem to do without much thought. While I am not here to take a stance on pro-life or pro-choice, I do want to shed light on how hard the decision is for a woman to make. In Vernette's case, it was a choice that would stay with her for the rest of her life.

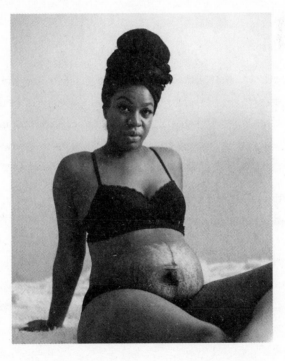

"How do you find atonement when you harbor guilt for a choice made in your teens?" I asked her.

"I knew very early in motherhood that I wanted to be intentional about my healing process after my early termination at sixteen. I struggled with the fact I took life from my own body. I felt empty and ashamed," Dr. Vernette admits.

"As I began to develop a more intimate relationship with Jehovah, this seed was planted in my heart. I wanted to give back. It became more and more clear that I would carry life for another. The puzzle pieces began to come together and even in the present day, postpartum, God continues to call on me to be a vessel for the goodness of humanity. He is full of miracles. He has truly blessed me."

*I feel complete.*

Dr. Vernette was matched with a couple in Israel and her journey began. She traveled between Georgia and California, underwent time-consuming evaluations and doctor appointments, but through the entire process, she remained positive. Then, in January of 2018, she got the news that she was pregnant.

Dr. Vernette chose to stay very open about her journey. She posted about it on her Instagram account and kept her children in the know about what was happening. "Was everyone understanding?" I asked her one day. She told me they weren't, but she understood why they didn't understand.

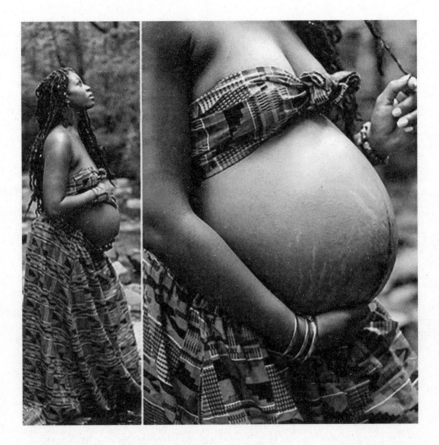

# Surrogacy in Real Life

Surrogacy is already a hard concept to grasp for most. Many women claim they could not carry a baby for nine months only to hand it over to another family. It is even more unheard of in the Black community. In fact, the first African American mother to give birth by surrogacy was Anna L. Johnson on September 19, 1990. Her case was controversial for many of the same reasons that most women say they couldn't become surrogates—Anna bonded with her baby and didn't want to give the child to the intended parents. Anna ended up losing a court case and parental rights to the child.

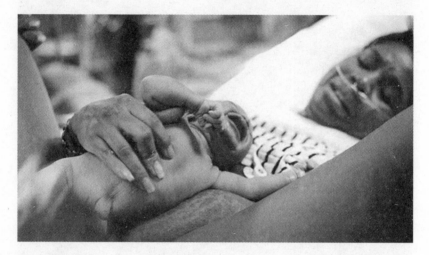

For those that aren't familiar with surrogacy, there are two types: traditional (which uses the mother's egg) and gestational surrogacy (the mother carries embryos only). Vernette had an embryo transfer, which is nonsurgical and noninvasive. A catheter is used to implant the embryo on the lining of the uterus, and from there the mother is put on bed rest for up to twenty-four hours for implantation to occur. The uterus will need to accept the embryos and a successful pregnancy is hopefully confirmed ten days later.

Like in Anna's case, Dr. Vernette gave birth to twin babies, neither of which carried her genes. In fact, Baby A was born with blond hair and Baby B with reddish hair. Each of the babies belonged to one of their respective fathers. After birth, when asked if she wanted to hold the babies, Dr. Vernette initially declined.

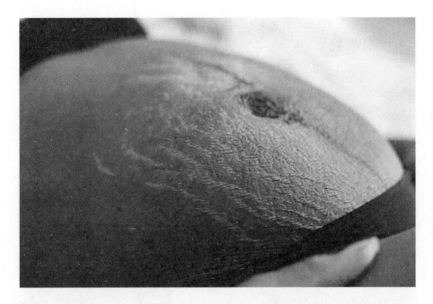

For Dr. Vernette, she had come to terms with the surrogacy process well before pregnancy even took place. Surrogacy isn't a flash thought. It takes much mental examination, preparation, and assurance to properly transpire.

# #THISISPOSTPARTUM

What's postpartum like after surrogacy? Dr. Vernette says:

> Outside of the occasional mood swing, I have been able to rest and take time to ease back into my routine of life— parenting two school aged littles, working with my patients to improve their well-being, investing in self-care practices, and doing life with my tribe. This is how I am built—to "do" life.

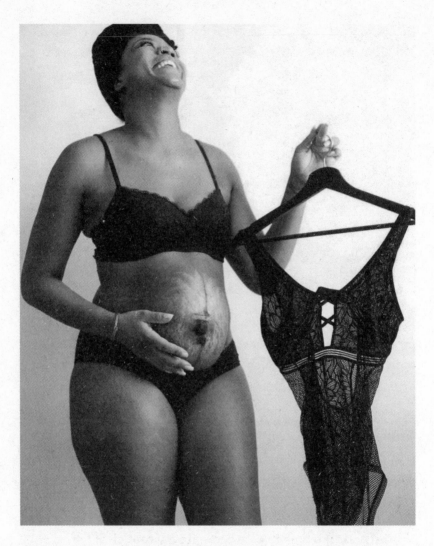

Dr. Vernette expresses that she is grateful to be able to spend time with the new fathers and their surro twins before they return home to Israel. The goodbye process has been longer and more intimate than most because the amazing fathers are staying in town for a month postdelivery. Their extended stay and openness to bond more has allowed their relationship to continue to grow into a family.

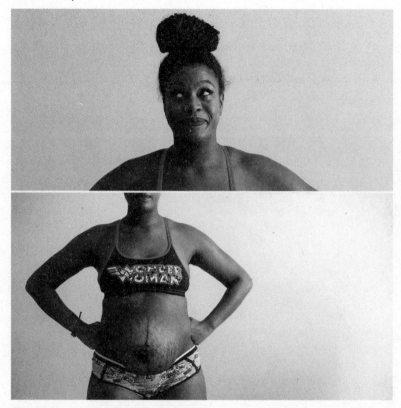

What's next for Dr. Vernette?

"I will continue to free flow," Dr. Vernette says.

> In my world, nothing is impossible. My mind is always at work and I am in the process of rebranding myself. I believe this experience has opened many conversations that empower women to soar in their greatness and I want to focus my brand on empowering women through holistic self-care practices

such as guided meditation, energy work, and movement therapy like Pilates and Yoga.

*It is important to highlight what pregnancy and postpartum looks like for all mothers, even surrogate ones. Birth is an initiation.*

*To learn more about Dr. Vernette, you can visit her website at DrVernette.com.*

# Chapter Twenty-Three

# How Sis Got Her Groove Back

*I just think, as women, we have to give ourselves room to be individuals. So when a woman makes a decision for herself, we as women shouldn't set those hardcore boundaries for another woman. Just like we don't want men setting hardcore boundaries for us.*

—Jada Pinkett Smith

**This could arguably be the** second most important chapter in our guidebook. Here's the thing. Pregnancy lasts for roughly ten months. Your labor and delivery can continue for any time period between twenty-four hours to three days—this is a very vague estimate. As you read in the previous chapters, your postpartum period can carry on for a year or two after your baby is born. After all of these processes, you are still going to have to show up for you. After pregnancy, labor, delivery, breastfeeding, and postpartum, you will still have to wake up every single morning, take a deep breath, and remember that you, Sis, you deserve it all. You are still a woman. I could not conceive writing this book without bringing our time together to a close by affirming just how powerful and wonderful you are. I needed to let you know this. I want you to feel this deep within your spirit because it took me many years to discover that I was still a person after becoming a mother.

One of the important factors of my inner drive to continue my platform, *Black Moms Blog*, is to help mothers understand that they are not in this mamahood gang alone. I believe that by using my own motherhood journey as my reference point, making note of the times I felt isolated, confused, stressed, and out of my own body, I could write about these occurrences and hopefully save at least one mama from the inner conflict of feeling like she just was not good enough. Good enough. What does that even mean? Believing that you have to be "good enough" as a mother is the mentality that you are never allowed to have any days off. It means that you wake up every morning with a smile on your face and show up for each and every person in your family and your life, including your friends, bosses, and companions, before you determine that it is necessary to show up for yourself.

It means taking that line, "sweatpants, hair tied, chillin with no makeup on" entirely too literally and forgetting that you can still adorn yourself, wear sexy lingerie, and be drop-dead gorgeous—even with your stretch marks. Drake was wrong about something. Your outer appearance, no matter if you are dressed down or dressed up, isn't when you are the prettiest. When your attitude and confidence, your self-love, is shining bright is when you are the most stunning. There is absolutely nothing wrong with remembering who you are. If you have not found Her yet before becoming a mother, you will certainly discover Her after childbirth.

# Be Honest with Yourself and Your Loved Ones

It is a gift and a curse to be a Black woman. Our melanin, our resilience, our sheer determination to get things done sets us apart. At the same time, the Black woman is the most unprotected person on this earth. We have to stand up, shout, and demand to be heard, only to be then classified as an Angry Black Woman. Your postpartum time is an extremely crucial period for you to remember to use your voice. You do not have to appear stronger than you are. If you are hurting, say that. If you feel depressed, speak on it. If you are not in the mood for sex with your partner, even after your medical provider has given you the green light, simply say, "Baby, I am not in the mood." A major step in getting your groove back is leaning into that community we spoke of in the previous chapters. You will find that more people around you want to help you than not.

Before asking for help, you must be honest with yourself and really determine how it is that you feel. One way you can do this is by keeping a postpartum journal. You can write out your daily emotions and write letters to yourself. I learned about the importance of journaling through Queen Afua's Sacred Woman's Rites of Passage program. Through her program, we kept womb journals, and while it was uncomfortable at first, I learned how to speak to myself, more specifically to my womb, in a loving way. In speaking to my womb, I was thanking myself for the hard work I had accomplished and giving praise to the strength my womb had shown in carrying my daughter. Journaling can help you process emotions and practice communicating your words properly to ask for what you need. If you answer, "I am fine" every time someone asks you how you are doing after having your baby, you are not going to receive a lot of support if you are actually not fine. Remember, Sis, you had the baby. Not your friends. Not your family. Not your partner. This is not the time to be passive aggressive with your needs and wants. Speak up.

## Health and Wellness Are Vital

I did a poll in one of *Black Moms Blog*'s community support groups and I asked the women, "How did you get your groove back after giving birth?" Surprisingly, more than 80 percent of the answers correlated their positive outlook on self after becoming a mom with how much time they put into working out and losing the baby weight. I tread lightly here. We talked earlier about how a snapback is not realistic and is not anything we should strive for. We should always be looking forward, not backward. Even still, to deny that health is wealth would be nonsensical. So what do you do to mind your weight? When you are breastfeeding, you may feel your energy level depleted, and in turn may think that eating more food will give you more energy and increase your breast milk. Instead of eating more, eat right. Choose highly nutritious foods and follow a manageable diet, not a crash diet. In *No Excuses!: The Power of Self-Discipline*, Brian Tracy says that a healthy diet is more successful than a fanatical diet. While you may lose weight in the beginning, fanatical diets are nearly impossible to keep up with. Create a meal plan that works well for your life and your schedule so that you can easily integrate it into your routine.

What about exercise? According to experts, only thirty minutes of exercise is needed every day to maintain your health. After having a baby, it is important not to incorporate any new types of working out that you did not do prior to your pregnancy or during your pregnancy without first consulting your health care provider. Your provider will give you the thumbs up to start back your fitness routine. Exercise can be intimidating if you have never done it. I say this from experience. It took three years for my post-baby-weight to really settle into my body. I gained nearly thirty pounds and my petite 130-pound figure quickly escalated to a hefty 160 pounds. Pregnancy did not knock me down, but motherhood took its toll. I joined a local fitness class to build my stamina and increase my cardio. Once I was comfortable with the idea of working out, I was able to work out in the gym alone. To meet certain fitness goals, I eventually invested in a personal trainer. In six months, I felt like I was in better shape than I had ever been. I felt sexy and confident because of it. Working out was a main contributing factor for getting my groove back. I no longer looked in the mirror and disliked what I saw. Ultimately,

I learned when it came to weight loss that it was not about what anyone else saw when they looked at me—it was how I felt when I looked at me. That was when I knew my habits had to change.

Some ways to incorporate exercise after childbirth are by first starting light. Purchase a jogging stroller so that you can take your baby with you. Even though it is called a jogging stroller, you can definitely start off with a brisk walk until you build up your stamina to jog or run. You can also join a local mom's group that meets up to work out or walk together. It is always easier when you have a support group. Remember the African proverb: If you want to go fast, go alone. If you want to go far, go together. The same notion applies in this scenario. Your goal in losing baby weight is not to do it quickly, it is to focus on the long game— creating habits that you can maintain for a lifetime. If you are feeling insecure about working out with others right away, you can also browse YouTube. There are plenty of mommy workouts and baby yoga exercises you can do in the comfort of your own home. Working out with your infant is a great way to bond as well. They will supply all the laughs and the weight. Your baby is a great replacement for a dumbbell!

# Hire Out if You Are Able

Hey Sis, you do not always have to be Superwoman. One of the best parts of this modern world is that you can literally pay people to help you with your daily to-do list. It takes a village to raise a child...and sometimes you have to pay that village. If you are in a financial position to do so, consider hiring a cleaning company to come by twice a month to deep clean your home or fold laundry. The cleaning company may not clean the way your grandmother cleans, but I can guarantee it will bring you some peace to not keep putting off that growing pile of dirty clothes. You can also have your groceries delivered to your front door or hire a meal-planning service that can drop off weekly meals that take less than thirty minutes to cook. If you are a stay-at-home mother, hire a nanny to come give you a break for a few hours a week. Staying at home with your baby is a blessing but it can also be extremely overwhelming.

# The Stay-at-Home Mother Versus the Working Father/Partner

When I was pregnant with my daughter, I knew that I wanted to be a stay-at-home mother. I always saw myself smiling and happy, nails painted, hair done, and presentable. I thought that my partner and I would spend weekends as family time and visit museums and parks together with our daughter. I am not sure what television show I was watching that somehow had engraved that ideology into my mind, but my reality was far different from my expectation. My reality all those years ago was that most times my home was a mess, we did not eat enough vegetables at dinner, and if I was lucky, I found time to paint my nails once every six months. The things people take for granted, like walking to and from their car, I found myself craving. The joys of grocery shopping alone or peeing in peace seemed to be a thing of the past. Being a stay-at-home mom felt like being a married single mother. It is this ugly side that no one wants to talk about or discuss—this loneliness and bitterness that can destroy relationships and marriages when it comes to children.

Many people believe that because a woman decides to be a stay-at-home mother, all responsibilities outside of bills should fall on her. She should cook breakfast, lunch, and dinner. She is supposed to keep her home clean by washing dishes, doing laundry, and supervising busy children. She is never supposed to lose her cool when dealing with her children and she is required to educate and entertain them from the time they rise until they are asleep. She is also expected to (happily) show up sexually and emotionally for her partner. A stay-at-home mom should make sure that her husband is able to walk into his home, put his feet up, and not have to deal with the daily activities that come with having a household with children. What a job.

This *job* does not have any lunch breaks, no PTO, it comes without a paycheck, and there is not any five o'clock time stamp. It is constant, twenty-four hours a day, seven days a week, and is hardly as luxurious as most people have made it out to be in their minds. It rarely comes with a thank you, there are no yearly bonuses, and the real work is normally not seen by those who benefit from it the most. According to Fox News, stay-at-home mothers are worth an average of $117k per year—that is more than your standard lawyer.[19]

This is not all woe. Stay-at-home mothers, also known as SAHMS, love what they do. SAHMS are thankful to provide for their families and to be there for every waking moment of their children's lives. It really is a beautiful occupation. But I think I can speak for all stay-at-home moms when I say this: sometimes a little help is needed from our partners. Saying you need assistance from your partner does not make you ungrateful. In reality, no

19    www.foxnews.com/story/2008/05/08/study-stay-at-home-mom-worth-nearly-117000-year.html

one truly gets a real break. A working partner is not only obligated to pay the bills. A working partner is expected to also lend a helping hand. They are expected to volunteer to wash the dishes after Mom has cooked for their family. Your partner should still romance you and make you feel special. Your partner is expected to take on bedtime duties from time to time and commit to spending time with their family outside of the home. Your other parent is expected to provide balance and grace.

A paycheck does not equate to spousal support. Mortgage payments do not take the place of giving the overworked stay-at-home mom a few hours of peace once or twice a week. As the saying goes: *A happy wife is a happy life.* Take the money out of the equation. If your partner could no longer say, "I pay the bills," in what ways are they having a helping hand in your family?

## Questions to Ask Yourself

- Is my partner listening to my concerns without being objective?

- Is my partner open to giving me alone time while I am energized and not exhausted after already completing my daily duties?

- Is my partner being considerate of my daily needs and frustrations?

- Would my partner happily switch roles with me and do my job without complaint?

If you find yourself answering no to any of these questions, it may be time to reevaluate how strong your support system is within your family. As you continue this process of trying to get your groove back, your voice will be your biggest advocate, Sis. Do not be afraid to use it.

# Find a Therapist

The idea of therapy is taking on fewer frightening connotations in the Black community. We are finally grasping the importance of mental health and don't associate seeking professional help with being crazy. Think of it like this—do you proactively take your car to the shop for oil changes or do you wait until the lack of oil causes a much more severe problem? If you are smart, you have an oil change every three months for your vehicle. Think of therapy with the same mindset.

Have you noticed a consistent theme throughout your guidebook? It is me constantly telling you the importance of using your voice, Sis. A therapist will help you find your voice when you can't remember where you sat it down. They will help you connect your emotions to certain events or to a mentality so that you can improve. If you and your partner are struggling with communication after your baby is born, therapy or counseling can also be a step in the right direction. Anything that improves your mental health will help you to regain your groove.

# Reclaim Your Sensuality

Isn't it interesting that the one thing that got you into this position can now become your least favorite activity? I began this subtopic with the title: Reclaim Your Sex Appeal. I quickly changed it. The truth is, getting your groove back is not about sex. It is about you. Sex is like the sweet cherry on top of delicious homemade butter-pecan ice cream...the kind with the whole pecans, not the crumbled pieces. Sex is what happens after you have tapped back into your sensuality. In *Pussy: A Reclamation*, Regena Thomashauer passionately writes about how rediscovering her sensuality and reclaiming her pussy—she somehow manages to make you look at your own pussy in an elegant way—saved her womanhood.

> They had to learn to see me as a sensual woman who desired a full, passionate life—not just a mother whose best years were behind her and whose future was limited to caring for grandchildren and other family members.

Can you feel that, Sis? Reclaiming her sensuality was Regena's way of getting her groove back. After becoming a mother, our sensuality takes the biggest hit. Our four-inch heels turn into Nike slides. Our sexy lingerie becomes whichever T-shirt doesn't have throw-up on it. Makeup is a thing of the past. We just stop caring and we hide behind the claim of motherhood as the excuse. "I'm a mom now. I don't have time for that!" *Stop* telling yourself this. Our bodies look different and our time has been restructured, but you have time for any single thing that you put intentional effort into. Your sensuality is one of them.

There is a scene in *Sex in the City* where Charlotte looks at her pussy for the first time. She takes a mirror to explore herself and Carrie hilariously narrates the story of Narcissus, a notable figure from Greek mythology who died while gazing into a pool at his own reflection. He was so entranced with his own beauty, he could not pull himself away, not even to eat, sleep, or drink. He was obsessed. My point in telling you this is not to have you become narcissistic over your pussy but rather to learn to love her again. Appreciate her. Feel her. Smell her. Give your pussy a name and rediscover who she is after childbirth. Even if you had a C-section, rediscovering your pussy is essential to reclaiming your sensuality. In a survey done by *Vice* in 2014, 44 percent of a thousand women were unable to identify their vagina on a medical illustration of the female reproductive tract.[20] 60 percent could not identify their vulva. Learning your anatomy is not just scientific, it is your basic womanly right.

Discovering your body goes far beyond your pussy. It means relearning your new curves, lines, and grooves. Practice standing in front of the mirror naked. Light your candles, run a warm bath, and nurture yourself on a weekly basis. Stand in front of your mirror and watch as your hands massage oil deep into your skin. Learn to make love to yourself again by reawakening the nerves in your skin with physical touch. Your baby does not own your body or your breasts. They are yours and can still be explored for pleasure. Your body is your altar. Adorn Her properly. I suggest going through your nighttime pajamas and discarding anything that makes you feel frumpy. There is still a way to feel comfortable without wearing a T-shirt from 2008 with seven holes and bleach stains splattered throughout. Invest in pajamas that make you feel sexy and that fit your new body. Trying to squeeze back into your pre-baby clothes can be discouraging if you have not lost the weight and achieved the body size that you desire. The goal is to regain your love of your inner self first and your outer self, your physicality, next. Once you have conquered your sensuality, your sexuality will follow in tow. For my mamas

20    www.vice.com/en/article/ppaka8/way-too-many-women-dont-know-where-their-vaginas-are.

that are in a relationship, this will be a joyous occasion. I cried the first time I had sex after walking in my power. I intensely sobbed because I felt that I had never known my body in the way that I had learned before. If you are not in a relationship, this process can look a bit different but still be just as positive.

# Intimacy and the Single Mom: Three Ways to Survive the Dry Spell

Talking about sex as a mom blogger is always a jarring experience. We post our wholesome family photos, our beautiful polka-dot dresses and clean kitchens. We show pictures of our smiling children, but the one thing that made all this possible is the topic we are mostly quiet about. SEX. Say that three times out loud for me.

S E X

S E X

S E X

Now that we have gotten that out of the way, we can move on. Most single mothers can admit that sex is very rare, especially when you are raising an infant. I spent all of my teenage years waiting to get to a point to have sex as freely as I could only to become an adult and realize that there are *way* more factors involved that lead to the nitty-gritty. Sex becomes much more difficult after momhood takes over and even *more* difficult when... gasp! You are a mom with absolutely no partner in sight. This is not a conversation on morality. If anyone deserves intimacy on a regular basis, it is definitely the overworked and exhausted mother. But when there isn't a lover around to satisfy those needs or we're unable to have sex for other reasons, and Sis, you are just not choosing to get down like that, how do you survive the dry spell?

# Become More Intimate with Yourself

This is akin to our previous conversation about learning to reclaim your sensuality. Becoming intimate with yourself is a combination of regaining your sensuality and your sexuality. Sexuality does not always involve another person and can be completely accomplished on your own.

> I tried and I tried to avoid
> But this thing was happening
> Swallow my pride, let it ride
> And parted, but this body felt just like mine
> I got worried
> I looked over to the left
> A reflection of myself
> That's why I couldn't catch my breath
> —"Oops, Oh My," Tweet

You remember that song, Sis? Tweet gave us the manual for self-pleasure. She goes on to sing:

> I looked over to my left
> Mmm, I was lookin' so good I couldn't reject myself
> I looked over to my left
> Mmm, I was feelin' so good I had to touch myself

If you are looking for some intimate pleasure and it is just you and your ten fingers, you can go the self-pleasuring route. I am hesitant to mention vibrators because if you are not being intimate on a regular basis, throwing a vibrator into the mix can keep you further away from human connection. A partner cannot pleasure you the way a Dickrunner 5000 can, right? So, I say proceed with extreme caution here. My advice would be to only pull out the vibes for special occasions and learn to enjoy your alone time on your own. If you have been lacking intimacy, everything just kind of goes numb down below. You forget what touch feels like and instead you find yourself groping around at lost body parts. Being intimate with yourself means making love to yourself. Take a note once again from our lesson on self-sensuality above. Set the mood. Start by just rubbing your fingers across your body and really try to connect with the sensation of touch. Once you become familiar with your body, it will be even easier to tell your future lover how to please you on their own.

# Channel That Energy into Another Space

Have you ever heard of thermodynamics? It is also known as the law of the conservation of energy. The first law of thermodynamics states that energy can neither be created nor destroyed; energy can only be transferred or changed from one form to another. The same law can be applied to sexual energy. I will be the first woman to admit that we probably think about intimacy more than a man does. For us, our lady parts don't give us away in public, so we have free range to daydream about that cute barista at Starbucks all day long if we want to. The truth is though, if you are not participating in any late-night action, it will hinder you more than help you to think about what could be happening but isn't all day long. Instead, find a way to channel that energy into another space. A few options to consider would be to pick up an exercise or a yoga class. Find a way to sweat it out in a different kind of way. Not only are you redirecting the energy, you are finding a way to get in shape and contribute positivity to your mental health.

# Go Ahead and Fully Commit

It may seem as if you have fully committed to not having sex, but unless you decide to actually *be* celibate, you are only taking a break until something good comes along. Celibacy is the act of abstaining from sexual relations until you accomplish a goal. This goal may be marriage or a journey through self-healing. Either way, even if the perfect partner does come along, you abstain from intimacy with this person until your goal has been obtained. Celibacy is no easy task, but it is something I recommend every woman try at least once in their life. Celibacy helps to reduce anxiety and can assist in rationalizing attraction. You learn the difference between lust and love. You are able to identify a person's true motives when sex is not on the table. You also learn just how strong you are mentally when you put a pleasurable task on the back burner while you consciously fix some inner battles with yourself. During your celibacy, it does not mean that you cannot date. It only means that you are dating without sex. It is possible. Journal through your hard days. Learn to manifest what you truly desire. You got this.

# Here Is the Greatest Secret: You Do Not Have to Get Your Groove Back. It Is Time to Discover a New You

Becoming a mother is a pure symbol of courage. Being a Black mother in this world is taking a stand. You are committed to changing the narrative around what people think when they see Black mothers. You picked up a copy of this book which means that you are intentional about breaking generational curses and have decided to have a healthy pregnancy, childbirth, and to walk into motherhood with your shoulders back and your head held high. Every time a woman gives birth, she is recreating her legacy and furthering her ancestral heritage. You did that. My hope in writing *Oh Sis! You're Pregnant!* was to not only celebrate Black motherhood but to also create a safe space for *us*. I know how it feels to be the lonely Black mother at play dates or to be judged by your doctor because you are young and presumably single. I get what it feels like to have to tell your mother that, even though you love her, it will stress you out to have her in the delivery room. I completely understand what it looks like to have to find yourself again after having a baby. These topics are just as important as the conventional information you find in most baby books—but this valuable knowledge is unique to the Black motherhood experience. I realized through writing these pages that we really haven't lost anything as much as we are discovering a new path, a new woman, a new us. My daughter has been by my side through this entire process. I told her, "I hope you follow through this guidebook if you ever decide to have children in your future." I am doing this not only for us but for the generations that come after us. For so long, all we have had to rely on for pregnancy advice are books like *What to Expect* and the Mayo Clinic guides. While these are important, there is much of the conversation that is disregarded.

There is no going back, Sis. You do not have to find something you dropped or left off elsewhere. You do not have to go back and pick up the pieces, fit into those old jeans, or even try to keep up with the same schedule you had before becoming a mother. That is an outdated version of yourself. Now, you have become someone else. You are a mother, but most importantly you are a new woman. I hope through the pages of this guidebook you have discovered new ideas, you have found joy, laughter, and taken some self-accountability. I pray that you pass this book on through your friendship circles, to your family members, and suggest it to the random Black pregnant woman you see while grocery shopping or playing with your kids in the park. I hope this book sparks a conversation in your life that leads to your developing a deeper relationship with your mother. I hope it brings your family closer together because your husband or partner reads it with you and learns how to become a better support system. This is *The Ultimate Guide to Black Pregnancy and Motherhood*. May you be blessed. May you be loved. May you become all the things that you need and more. Welcome to the super-dope tribe of Black motherhood.

# Acknowledgements

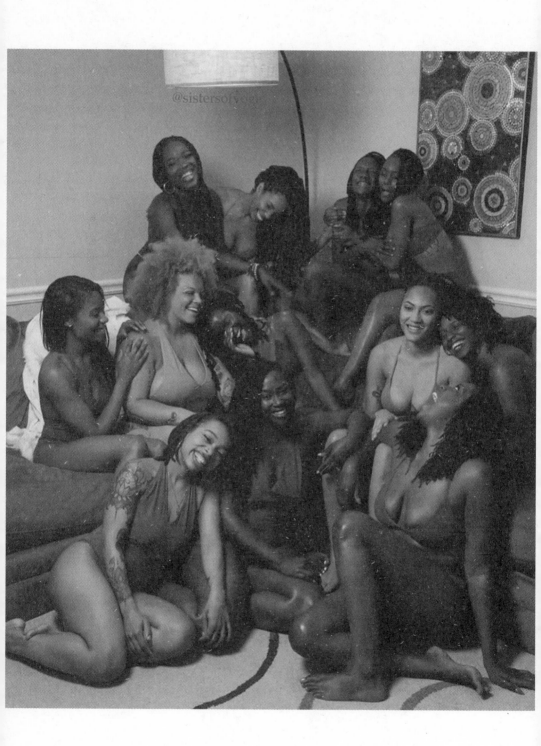

**Of all the words I** prepared to write for *Oh Sis, You're Pregnant!*, writing my acknowledgements made me the most nervous. There are so many people who poured into this book because there are so many people that have poured into me—not just in the course of me writing *Oh Sis*, but those who have given me encouragement, heartbreak, disbelief, and love throughout my life. All parts of those emotions went into these pages, so it is only right that I give thanks to all in its entirety.

As when I rise and the same for when I rest, my very first and final thanks will always be given to The Most High, Jehovah God. Thank you for all the things, many of them which I could never publicly express thanks for, but for this book I will say thank you for instilling in me the confidence that I am special and that I was placed here with a real purpose. Thank you for giving me a voice that has continuously served as a positive representation of the most Divine spirit on this earth, the Black mother. We are made in Your image.

One of the most special parts of writing *Oh Sis* is that my daughter has been present for the majority of the process. She has watched me spend many hours researching, typing, interviewing, and pushing myself to the limit to make sure that what I created with the hopes of it being the ultimate pregnancy guide for Black women held true to its promise. I told her that if she decides to have children in her adulthood, I wanted this guidebook to lead her through a healthy and stable pregnancy. To my lovely daughter, Kamryn Amelia Banks, thank you for choosing me to be your mother. As you say to me, perfection is not real, but baby girl, you are as close to perfect for me as you could ever be. I am so excited to watch you grow up.

I would like to thank my mother. I did not understand love until I became a mother to my own daughter, and only then could I fully understand the sacrifices my mother had made for my brother and me. My mother is one of the softest and simultaneously most fierce women I know. For years, I ran from her fierceness and tried to calm her waters, but her strength rubbed off on me as well as her softness. She was my example of feminine nature and showed me what unconditional love really looked like. My mother spoiled me in kindness and endearment. Because of her, I possess the ability to always be aware of gentleness when sharing space with my own daughter. This book came through our bloodline, Mama. So much gratitude to my ancestors: Nellie Jones, Carrie Jackson, and Wanda "Katie" Edwards.

Ase'.

I want to thank each and every woman that has shared their personal stories with me. Some in close sister circles. Others through *Black Moms Blog*. Some of these stories were passed to me through tears, laughter, disappointment, and embarrassment. That section on hemorrhoids definitely came from a sister who couldn't use the bathroom! As she expressed her discomfort to me over the phone, I made a note to add that into this book— because I knew she was not the only one who experienced that pain. It was important to me that every woman felt seen. I want to thank each woman who showed up in vulnerability in front of my camera to let me photograph their bodies. Some of those photo shoots were therapy sessions for both of us. This book is composed of so many stories I have been graciously gifted by the women around me. I am thankful to have put them into words. Thank you all for trusting me to present your most intimate moments to the world in a way that you still feel protected. A special thank you to Vernette for allowing me to tell her story of surrogacy time and time again. You are powerful, Sis.

Thank you to *Black Moms Blog* and all the opportunities I have been provided through your outlet. I created an entity that has become much bigger than me. It deserves its own acknowledgement. *Black Moms Blog* helped me define my voice, led me into a space of healing—at first for mothers and then for women—and ultimately became a masterful connector for me to so many women around the world. I am forever grateful.

Thank you to a few special people who provided me a safe space to write when I hit blockages. I was able to escape home for days at a time, lock myself away, and write to my heart's content. Thank you to the women who have mentored me over the years. To Courtney and Phnewfula, I love you both for believing in my book cover fiercely when I was discouraged from using my own photography. The belief in all of my close friends carried me over this finish line. Thank you to Alexandre Keto. It is an honor to have your artwork in *Oh Sis*. Thank you to my publishing company who signed me and sat patiently as I finished this book. This was a manifestation. I said I wanted to write a book, and a few weeks later I had an email from my publishing house offering a contract. Look at Gawd.

To Agatha, Tracie, Krystal, Heather, and Aiyana, your contributions to Oh Sis are going to help so many women. Thank you.

Last but not least, I want to say thank you to each experience in my life that may have seemed negative at the time, but which caused me to grow. Because of these situations, I was able to write about how to deal with the adversity of being a single

Black woman with a child. I was able to write about how I healed through the broken relationship that put me there. I was able to speak openly about how I found out how to love myself again as a woman and not just a mother. I reclaimed my body, my spirit, and my mind from changing friendships, bad relationships, and insecurities. I overcame so that I could teach another woman how to do the same. Oh my Goddess! Thank you for growth!

# About the Author

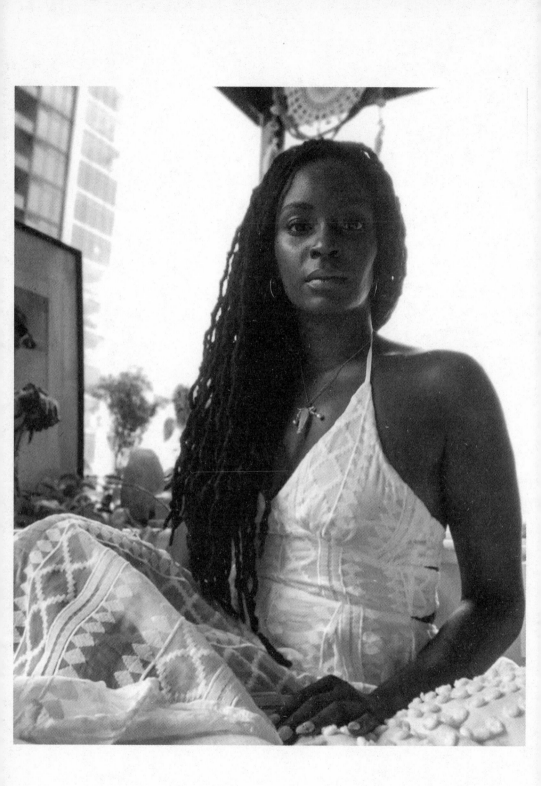

**Shanicia Boswell is a woman** of many talents. She is a friend, a mother, a serial entrepreneur, an author, and a facilitator of women's healing circles. She is most widely known for being the creator of Black Moms Blog, a global collaborative platform that discusses parenting, culture, and lifestyle from a Black mom's point of view. Her initiative has not only served her online community of more than half a million women but has created many social movements such as the Menstrual Drive and Period Party, which collects menstrual items for women's homeless shelters and educates women and young girls on their periods and how the foods we eat and products we use affect our bodies. Through Black Moms Blog, Shanicia Boswell also created the Nursathon, a conference aimed to increase the statistics on breastfeeding in mothers of color through education, awareness, and resources. In 2020, the Nursathon sponsored two women through their doula certification training. Her other businesses include a retreat company, The Self Care Retreats, and her photography business, Yeyo Photography. Her daughter Kamryn LLC'd her very first business, Sunshine Honey Books, a book series based around her life as a precocious and explorative child.

As a sought-out expert and pioneer for Black motherhood and self-care, Shanicia has been featured on major television syndications such as the OWN Network and CNN's HLN Weekend Express as a guest moderator on Saturday mornings. She has spoken at numerous conferences on millennial Black motherhood, ways to better communicate with our children, and diversity training in adolescence. Shanicia is a contributor to the parenting section of the New York Times and Washington Post, as well as writing for Parents, Huffington Post, and other major platforms.

To learn more about Shanicia, you can visit her website ShaniciaBoswell.com. To learn more about Black Moms Blog, visit BlackMomsBlog.com. To purchase Kamryn's book, visit SunshineHoneyBooks.com.

**You can follow Shanicia on her social accounts below:**

**Instagram:** @shaniciaboswell and @blackmomsblog

**Facebook:** @blackmomsblog

**Twitter:** @blackmomsblog

**Website:** www.shaniciaboswell.com
and www.blackmomsblog.com

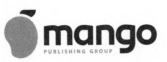

Mango Publishing, established in 2014, publishes an eclectic list of books by diverse authors—both new and established voices—on topics ranging from business, personal growth, women's empowerment, LGBTQ studies, health, and spirituality to history, popular culture, time management, decluttering, lifestyle, mental wellness, aging, and sustainable living. We were recently named 2019 *and* 2020's #1 fastest growing independent publisher by *Publishers Weekly*. Our success is driven by our main goal, which is to publish high quality books that will entertain readers as well as make a positive difference in their lives.

Our readers are our most important resource; we value your input, suggestions, and ideas. We'd love to hear from you—after all, we are publishing books for you!

Please stay in touch with us and follow us at:

> Facebook: Mango Publishing
>
> Twitter: @MangoPublishing
>
> Instagram: @MangoPublishing
>
> LinkedIn: Mango Publishing
>
> Pinterest: Mango Publishing
>
> Newsletter: mangopublishinggroup.com/newsletter

Join us on Mango's journey to reinvent publishing, one book at a time.